A Dog Lover's Guide

to

CANINE MASSAGE

A Dog Lover's Guide

to

CANINE MASSAGE

by

Jody Chiquoine
RN, MSN, FNP, CRRT

&

Linda Jackson
Lic.Ac, MAcOM, MEd

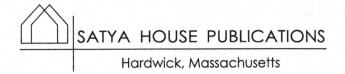

SATYA HOUSE PUBLICATIONS
Hardwick, Massachusetts

Disclaimer

This book is written for dog owners and is not meant to replace proper diagnosis and treatment from a qualified veterinarian. It is intended to compliment proper veterinary care and/or care from other canine professionals.

Massage and stretching should always be done with caution and any body work with dogs is taken exclusively at one's own risk. The authors assume no liability for use of canine massage and/or stretching techniques described in this book.

ISBN: 978-0-9729191-7-3

Library of Congress Control Number: 2008931684

Photo Credits:
All photos © 2008 by Linda Jackson with the following exceptions:
Pages 73 and 74 photos by Sandra Murley
Page 90 photo by Cris Raymond
Page 91 photo by Julie Murkette
Page 105 photos by Amy Fish
Page 107 photo by Nora Adelman

TABLE OF CONTENTS

Acknowledgements   7
Canine Massage Introduction   9
How to Use This Book   11

Chapter 1   Body Language of Your Dog   13

Chapter 2   What Is Massage?   17
             The Benefits of Massage   18
             How to Touch   20
             The Do's and Don'ts of Massage   21
             Contraindications or When Not to Do Massage   22
             Teaching Your Dog to Receive a Massage   23

Chapter 3   Strokes — The Gift We Give Our Dogs   27
             Effleurage   28
             Petrissage   30
             Skin Rolling   31
             Compression   32
             Vibration   34
             Shaking   35
             Tapotement (Percussion)   36
             Friction   37
             Wringing   38
             Rocking   39

Chapter 4   Canine Anatomy in a Nut Shell   41

Chapter 5   Stretches   69

Chapter 6   A Massage Routine   77
             The Bullet Version of the Massage Sequence   84

Chapter 7   Frequently Asked Questions   85

Chapter 8   Common Dog Groups:
             Their History, Stress Areas and Massage Emphasis   90
             Dog Group Classifications   91

Glossary of Terms   101

About the Authors   105

Bibliography   109

Acknowledgements

The task of completing *A Dog Lover's Guide to Canine Massage* has truly been the work of many — both canine and human. We would like to thank those who have helped shape this book into reality.

First and foremost, gratitude is given to our dogs who have served as teachers. They have helped us to improve our skills and have shared with us the depth of the canine-human bond. We are humbled by their tolerance and patience. These canine friends continue to foster our growth and our endless gratitude is wrapped in every stroke, stretch and kiss! They have deeply touched our hearts.

Over the past five years we have had many participants in our canine massage classes. These individuals have participated in the ever-evolving course design and have offered valuable feedback for improving programs. They have strongly encouraged us to write this book and have provided the many photographic opportunities that are included in these pages. We are humbled to watch them learn canine massage and then at the end of each class, witness the intense bond when they offer their canine companion a relaxing massage.

We would like to thank those health professionals who choose to work as part of a collaborative team. It is this teamwork and collaboration that helps owners offer their dogs a full and happy life. Whether veterinarian, rehabilitation therapist, dog trainer or caretaker, it is that quality of care and love that contributes so very much to our pets.

We would like to hugely thank Julie Murkette for sharing our vision of dogs and Satya House Publishing for making this dream a reality.

Many enormous heartfelt thanks to our friend, dog lover and editor extraordinare, Cris Raymond. We will be forever grateful for the endless hours she (and her dog Chiara) spent with us with pencils, her giant dictionary and many cups of her famous ginger tea. In shaping our ideas into words, Cris is always honest, kind and relentless. Thank you, thank you, thank you.

From Jody:

Thank you to my beloved Great Pyrenees Remy for teaching me to always have Courage. I wrote this for you.

"Thank you" does not begin to express the gratitude I feel for my husband, Tim. His support, fantastic ideas, endless patience and caring is beyond words. Without these, the book would not have been possible.

To my late mother who loved creatures great and small and inspired me when I felt like quitting.

To my father I give thanks for teaching me the quality of tenacity and the belief that anything is possible.

From Linda:

Foremost I thank my daughter Kate, for her humor, her willingness to walk the dogs when I couldn't, for feeding back to me what I have always taught her — that anything is possible — and for her trust in me that I could indeed write a book.

Endless gratitude goes to my teachers — my dogs, Gypsy, Sachi and Romeo — for allowing me to stop writing in mid-sentence to do massage so that what I was expressing was accurate. I owe you a lifetime of massage.

And of course, many thanks go to my parents who, from an early age, instilled determination in me. And thanks to my sister Carol, who takes me away scuba diving every May, where pens and pencils simply aren't appropriate, but having fun is!

Canine Massage Introduction

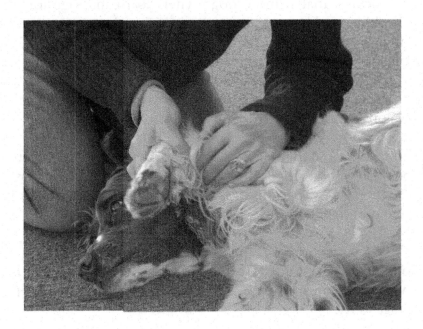

Dogs are our link to paradise.
They don't know evil or jealousy or discontent.
To sit with a dog on a hillside on a glorious afternoon is to be back in Eden,
where doing nothing was not boring – it was peace.

— Milan Kundera

The importance of canine massage is reflected in the fact that by offering regular massage to our pet companions, we can identify problems earlier and visit the veterinarian sooner. As a result of regular massage, it is clear that our dogs hold less stress in their muscles and are injured and sick less often.

When we do massage, we become the first detectives of problems whether it is a muscle knot, a lump, an embedded tick or pain. The more we massage, the more sensitive our hands and fingers become in detecting imbalances. Since our hands learn the feel of a healthy body, they can feel when a problem arises. We become alert to any changes in tissue, abnormal responses or to warning signals that may require professional attention.

Through regular massage, owners create both a maintenance and preventive health program. Injuries are less frequent as the body relaxes and stress is eased. Massage helps with the relaxation process and reduces muscle tightness.

Dogs live in the moment. When anxious, they might snap or bite and then it is over and they are ready to play again. Dogs don't hold stress in their bodies the same way that people do. They release their stress more easily and more quickly than humans do.

From our own positive experiences, we began to explore the concept of teaching massage to dog owners. We believe that if more dog owners learn massage for their dogs, both parties would be healthier and happier. Twice a year we teach a canine massage program to dog owners and their dogs. We watch the bonds deepen between people and their canine companions. In one brief day, people feel confident that they have valuable beginning tools to use at home to actively participate in the health and well being of their dogs. They walk away with skills to massage their dogs. In every class, we end the day deeply moved by the closeness that develops in an already close relationship.

From working with people and their dogs, we are convinced of the necessity of massage for health and well being. It is more than a pleasurable indulgence. It is a necessity for complete health. Massage is actually easy to learn. It is only the practice of it that becomes a challenge as it does take time on a regular basis to master the techniques and feel confident in the flow.

Although this book serves as a guide to canine massage, the real teacher is your dog. You will find that he will teach you all you need to know and all you need to do is just to listen and have the courage to try.

— Jody Chiquoine and Linda Jackson

HOW TO USE THIS BOOK

*The gift which I am sending you is called dog
and is in fact the most precious and valuable possession of mankind.*
— Theodorius Gaza "Canis Laudatio"

Welcome to *A Dog Lover's Guide to Canine Massage!*

Below are some ideas on how to use this book. It is our hope that after you have read this book, you will apply the information learned on your dog and that you both enjoy the benefits!

Read the entire book and then go back and use the techniques on your dog chapter by chapter. The book is organized so that after Chapter 1, each chapter builds on the previous chapter until the entire massage routine is completed.

Throughout the book are sections labeled Workbook Section. This is an opportunity for you to reflect on the material presented through directed questions and often includes exercises for you to practice. In the chapters on Strokes, Anatomy and Stretching, you will find Workbook Sections throughout the chapter at the end of important pieces of information.

This book was planned as a guide to our massage trainings, hence, the workbook style. If you are a licensed massage therapist who includes dogs in your professional practice, our hope is you will find this book an invaluable guide to your work.

Chapter One

Body Language of Your Dog

The reason a dog has so many friends is that he wags his tail rather than his tongue.
— Anonymous

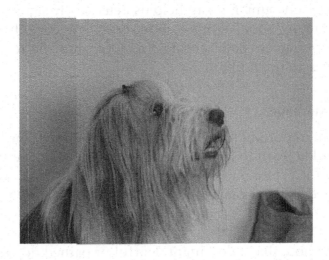

What Is Your Dog Telling You?

Dogs cannot communicate with words. Instead, they express themselves by eye movement, tail carriage, walking pattern, body stance, ear placement and lip motion. Dogs communicate to us and each other primarily through their bodies. This is called body language.

In a recent university study, dogs tested higher than any other animal, including monkeys, on their ability to "read" human body language. There is no doubt that they read body language much better than humans do.

Most of us have wondered how our dogs know when we are taking them on a hike on Saturday rather than going to work. They know when the weekend arrives by shrewdly watching the donning of old jeans and sweatshirt rather than blazer and slacks. However, the real clincher is the shoes. When you trade in your Gucci's for the well-worn sneakers or hiking boots, your dog knows the leash is next!

Dogs are perhaps the most observant of all species. While you may believe your dog to be sleeping, he is often listening or perceiving your most subtle energy shift. Just notice his ears while he sleeps. For example, the way you move in your chair just before finishing your newspaper means that the next activity is that his dinner will be prepared. The dog sits up, wags his tail, comes and nudges you and trots toward the kitchen. You wonder how he could know that you have finished the paper. A dog would be the ultimate poker player because he never misses a nuance.

Why is this ability to read body language almost a spiritual intuitive capability that is so developed in dogs? In the wild, from which all dogs derive, survival depended on this "sign" reading. Approaching a dominant leader in the wrong way could trigger an attack. Inability to "read" the weakness of prey animals could result in starvation. So dogs, as descendants of wolves, developed these keen senses.

How Does Body Language Matter to Us?

A thorough understanding of body language can help protect us and our pet from aggressive or assertive dogs that we encounter. It can help us detect early signs of worry and sickness in our dog. There are many books written about body language. In addition, many dog training manuals have chapters dedicated to this topic and the reader is encouraged to explore more on this fascinating subject.

Body Language and Massage

Body language plays an important role with massage as we watch the dog's response to our touch. Some dogs quickly learn to love being touched and will gleefully place themselves on the spot you or they select for massage. Other dogs initially may not like the touch with intent that is associated with massage and will look away, anxiously lick their lips and lower their head.

It is most important to note that a dominant, fearful or pained dog may nip if stressed. A dominant dog may be difficult to position and not wish to lie or settle, especially to lie on his side. He may also be verbal and growl when his paws, ears, head or tail are touched. Massage should be relaxing and fun. Instead, respond to what the dog will allow you to do. For example, initially massage a small part of the dog's body such as neck or shoulders and limit the time to one to three minutes.

Fearful or shy dogs may cower away, pull the tail between the legs and look at you with "side" eyes. Side eyes occur when the dog does not look directly at you but looks sideways with only his eyes turned toward you. The look can be intense or fearful and he may move his eyes from looking at you to looking away from you. Use caution if your dog looks at you with side eyes because he may nip or bite with no warning. In this case, you may want to begin with gentle petting and very subtly begin to increase the pressure. Try not to change your intent as the energy shift may frighten the dog until he becomes accustomed to this new approach.

As with the dominant dog, begin with short sessions of one to three minutes, end before the dog becomes alarmed and fearful and limit the size of the area being treated.

Dominant or fearful/shy dogs will do well to work with a trainer, behaviorist or veterinarian. Aromatherapy, herbs and homeopathic treatments may also help. Dogs with pain should always be evaluated by a veterinarian so that the cause of the pain can be determined. Your veterinarian may prescribe additional modalities such as medication, acupuncture, chiropractic, hydrotherapy (swimming in a therapeutic pool) or seeking help from a certified canine rehabilitation therapist. Once the area of pain and cause are determined, begin your massage over parts that are not painful. Begin with a light touch and slowly and gradually deepen the pressure. Cryotherapy (heat and/or cold packs) applied to painful areas or trigger points may be beneficial. Laying on of hands (*see Chapter 3 Strokes*) also may be beneficial. Always begin with long, soft strokes over painful areas and carefully watch your dog's body language to avoid a nip or bite. Be especially careful to keep your face away from his face when working over painful areas.

Your dog can not say "ouch" but he may move away from your touch, his skin may twitch, he may stare at you or get up and leave. In any of these cases, the pressure is too hard and should be lightened and preceded by hot and/or cold packs.

Watching your dog's response to touch and his body language in response to you is one of joyful exploration. Most of us force our dog to learn our verbal language and we never take the time to learn his. Give your dog the gift of learning his language and communicating on his terms too. This learning will enhance your understanding, bonding and mutual trusting to its highest levels.

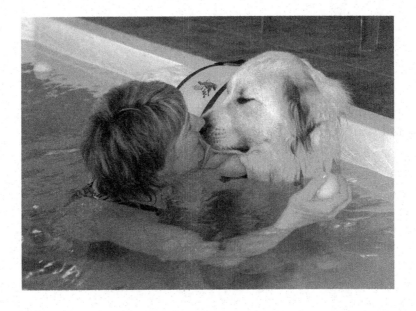

Workbook Section

1. Subtly observe your dog while he is lying still. What is he doing?

2. Lie on the floor with your dog, close your eyes and gently pet him for a period of time. What do you feel physically and emotionally?

3. Watch carefully as your dog approaches other dogs. What does his body language tell you?

4. Spend some time communicating with your dog without using words. What did your dog tell you? And what did you tell your dog?

Chapter Two

What Is Massage?

Massage must be simple.

— Plato

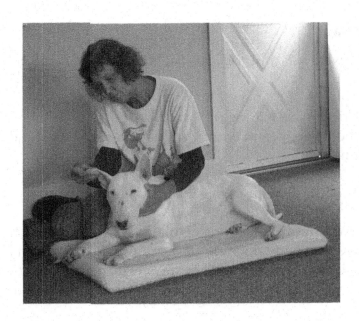

Massage has been part of the medical practices of many cultures for centuries. In the Orient and in India, massage still is part of the medical practices of these countries. In China, *Tui Na* (massage) uses manipulations to the soft tissue to improve range of motion and heal injury. In medical texts, Tui Na was used for specific areas of the body for healing and not as a general full-body massage. In Thailand, massage is done with stretching. In India, massage is part of Ayurvedic medicine used to cleanse the body of impurities. In Japan, acupressure and Shiatsu are the bodywork practices used both for healing as well as keeping the body in balance.

The massage most of us are familiar with is referred to as Swedish massage and the names of the strokes are in French. These names have been in use at least since the 1800s when the stroke names appeared in the *Proceedings of the German Society for Surgery*. Massage is manipulating the soft tissue in order to stimulate various physiologic responses. These mechanical actions involve pushing, pulling and friction. Massage is purposeful touch and, although simple, is not always easy to practice and perfect.

In our time, massage has been seen primarily as a pleasurable indulgence reserved for the wealthy. In the last 20 years, massage has been regaining its place as a healing, therapeutic modality as well as a pleasurable experience offered in spas around the world. To become a massage therapist now requires an extensive course of study, clinical training and a license to practice in most states. A growing number of massage therapists work therapeutically in professional and medical settings as well as at spa areas.

Massage, as a therapeutic tool, is now recognized within mainstream medical professions and is integrated more fully into hospital settings, physical therapy offices, chiropractic clinics as well as acupuncture practices. Also, massage is becoming more recognized in veterinary medicine. There are professionals in equine massage and canine massage in both veterinary clinics and rehabilitation settings. Many massage therapists are well trained and incorporate human and canine massage into their work. Massage is now clearly a solid part of healthcare and will only become more so.

The Benefits of Massage

> *Dogs are not our whole lives, but they make our lives whole.*
> — Roger Caras

You know from experience that massage not only feels good but it helps release tight muscles and assists you in finding your calm center especially after a stressful day. The same is true for dogs and all animals.

Here is a list of some of the benefits of massage:

- Massage relieves stress. When done regularly, it helps prevent the negative effects of stress. Of course dogs experience stress and although they don't seem to hold stress in their bodies the same way we do, stress, over time, can cause deeper long-term problems that require more serious intervention.

- Massage is soothing and comforting. Who doesn't need soothing and comforting? Consider times when your dog might need soothing or comforting.

- Massage calms the nervous system by giving repeated signals to the muscles to relax.

- Massage triggers the body's natural ability to heal itself from injury, strain, surgery and exhaustion. There are those times when we or our dog are injured, or perhaps even have had surgery. Massage is often the best therapy to assist in the healing process.

- Massage enhances circulation and stimulates muscles especially through petrissage, kneading and skin rolling *(see Chapter 3 Strokes)*. Massage assists the delivery of nutrients, oxygen and arterial blood components to the areas being massaged. Simply, this means improved overall health.

- Massage directly affects the autonomic nervous system for relaxation and mental calm.

- Massage is an effective tool to detect stiffness, pain, swelling, tension and in the long run can avoid costly complications from overlooked problems.

- Massage aids elimination of biochemical toxins as a result of improving circulation.

- Massage maximizes normal function of tissues, organs and bodily systems such as digestion, absorption of nutrients, elimination and the lymph system. Simply by the stress release and relaxation that massage produces, the entire body works more efficiently.

- Massage helps muscles function more efficiently by loosening restrictions as a result of misuse or over use of our muscles. We all know the pain created when we continue to work when exhausted. One example is working out too long or too hard at the gym, or when we take longer walks after a sedentary winter.

- Massage reduces the build-up of adhesions in the muscles that result from inflammation due to injury, surgery or trauma. Adhesions limit range of motion by shortening the muscles. We can feel adhesions as ropy areas in muscles surrounding an injury.

- Massage improves our dog's agility whether in play or competition because of its positive effect on stretch receptors, tendon apparatus, muscle fibers and fascia.

- Massage encourages relaxation of the tissues through aiding in more efficient functioning of the nerves and chemical changes in the body.

- Massage, through the friction strokes and stretching, creates a deliberate inflammatory response that in turn has the effect of "jump starting" the healing process. The resulting inflammatory responses inspire tissue repair in cases of injury and strain by calling forth the healing and energy cells of our body.

- Massage benefits include the reduction in symptoms of pain perception. Even though pain enables us to protect ourselves from greater damage, the reduction of pain also allows our body to heal properly.

- Massage softens and stretches the connective tissue that may impinge on nerves, thus relieving pain from pinched nerves.

- Massage normalizes a muscle tension pattern that restores a more normal resting length to shortened muscles that also reduces pressure on impinged nerves.

- Finally and perhaps most importantly, massage increases the physical and emotional bond between you and your companion canine.

WORKBOOK SECTION

1. What benefits have you experienced from massage?

2. What benefits do you think your dog will experience?

How to Touch

When doing massage, the quality of your touch is important. If you have had a massage from different therapists, then you probably know that there is some touch you like and some that you don't. The same holds true for your dog. If your touch isn't firm enough or too firm, your dog will not relax into the experience.

Compare the proper touch of massage to a hand shake. There are the handshakes that are limp, and those that are too forceful, like a vice grip. Then there is the handshake that feels firm and confident. The same is true of massage. A touch that is too light is unpleasant and has no intention behind it. Your dog will be confused and walk away or give you some signal that says he is not enjoying the experience.

A touch that is too forceful hurts. Your dog will let you know if you are hurting him. He will signal with his ears, his eyes, his posture and his tail. He may even growl or nip if the stroke is painful. He will struggle to get away from the experience.

The best touch is a firm and confident touch. This is the touch that has the intention of massage, which is to relax and soothe tired muscles. A firm and confident stroke communicates that you know what you are doing, has the purpose of massage and is a touch that feels safe and can be trusted. This is the touch that will teach your dog to relax with each stroke and enjoy the benefits of massage.

The Do's and Don'ts of Massage

The lists below are simple reminders of how to make the massage experience rewarding for both you and your dog.

DO's

- Wait for 30 minutes to an hour after strenuous exercise such as a long hike. Waiting allows the muscles, circulation and body temperature to return to normal. It also lets the excitement of the exercise settle so your dog will relax easier into a massage.

- Remove burrs, mud, ticks, dirt, etc. before beginning massage. Otherwise, the massage can embed such articles into the skin, which is unhealthy and can be extremely uncomfortable for both you and your dog.

- Work indoors. Although working outdoors might seem attractive, there are many distractions from noise, small wild animals and bugs. Working indoors provides an environment where distractions can be more under your control.

- Keep other pets away, as much as possible. Other pets can be a distraction until everyone knows what massage is about. If you have other dogs, they will generally wait their turn once they have experienced massage.

- Set the tone with a quiet environment, music and soft lighting.

- Begin with light strokes to warm an area and progress to deeper strokes. Beginning with deep strokes is like the forceful handshake. Without warming an area first with light strokes, the deeper strokes can hurt and actually do more harm than good.

- Talk softly to your dog during the massage. Dogs appreciate assurance during any massage and especially when you are beginning massage with him.

- Avoid massaging with long fingernails as they get in the way of effective massage strokes. Also avoid wearing heavy perfume. Your dog's keen sense of smell makes heavy perfume an unpleasant experience. Your dog would actually prefer your natural body odor.

- Pay attention to what your dog is communicating through his eyes, ears, tail, breathing or posture changes. He may be telling you that something you are doing is uncomfortable or that the session is over.

- Establish a schedule such as doing massage at the same time of day or days of the week. Dogs like routine and a set schedule is part of teaching your dog to receive a massage.

DON'TS

- Don't talk to someone else while doing massage. Your dog will sense your distraction and will likely move away.

- Don't speak loudly during massage. Loud tones, whether to your dog or to someone in another room, are certain to change the focus of the massage.

- Don't have loud music playing or distracting commotion around you. These activities change the intention and make it difficult for both you and your dog to focus.

- Don't smoke during massage. Smoking is a distraction that can injure your dog should hot ashes accidentally drop on him, and the smell of smoke is unpleasant.

- Don't work too quickly or forcefully. Massage is a time to relax. The slower and more focused your strokes, the easier it is for your dog to relax into the experience. If limited time is a factor, wait until you have the time to devote to a slow and relaxed pace.

- Don't ignore the contraindications of massage. The contraindications, when not to do a massage, are important so you don't worsen a condition.

Contraindications or When Not to Do Massage

Contraindications are situations, conditions and times when we should not do massage at all or we should wait until medical clearance is given from your veterinarian. There are two categories of contraindications, *absolute* and *local*. Absolute contraindications are those when massage is not advised because it could worsen a situation or condition, such as an infection. Local contraindications are those conditions in which massage can be given while avoiding an affected area or area in question.

Absolute Contraindications — Do Not Massage:

- If your dog has a fever, a temperature over 102°F. A good idea is to find out from your veterinarian what the normal temperature of your dog is, as normal can fall into a range among different breeds. Average is usually around 101°F.

- If your dog has just been seriously injured and is in shock, get to your veterinarian immediately. Do not attempt massage.

- If your dog has a viral disease such as distemper or influenza, especially in the acute stages of these conditions.

- If your dog has a skin problem of fungal origin such as ringworm, infectious diseases, pneumonia or bacterial skin diseases. Massage can make these conditions worse. Some skin diseases can be transferred from your dog to you.

- If your dog has tissue inflammation it can be worsened by massage.

- If your dog has diarrhea due to infection.

- If your dog has a serious injury or has had recent surgery, wait 48-72 hours.

Local Contraindications

- Avoid areas of cancerous tumors or cysts. It is unclear whether massage can spread cancerous growth, so avoiding the area is a good idea.

- Avoid open wounds or bleeding. If the wound has just happened, a veterinarian's attention is needed. Otherwise, avoid the area in order to let the healing happen without further injury or aggravation.

- Avoid acute trauma such as a torn muscle, broken bone or internal bleeding.

- Avoid the area of acute sprain or swelling. However, massage to the surrounding muscles can be relaxing and facilitate your dog's natural healing response.

- Avoid the abdominal area of a pregnant dog and pay attention to signals as to whether she wants massage or not.

- Avoid areas of acute arthritis. This is an inflammatory joint condition that can be aggravated or worsened with massage. Avoid massaging directly during acute flare-ups. Light massage is fine for relieving aches and stiffness when the arthritis is in the chronic stage.

TEACHING YOUR DOG TO RECEIVE A MASSAGE

No one appreciates the very special genius of your conversation as the dog does.
— Christopher Morley

Learning to relax is a learned skill and massage is a great way to teach, practice and experience the relaxation response. The more we practice, the easier it is to remain relaxed, even in the face of stressful situations. In 1975, Herbert Benson wrote a book called *The Relaxation Response* in which he introduced the idea that stress contributed to health problems and that relaxation increases our potential for self-healing. The advent of his ideas created an awareness of the value of meditation, yoga, stress-reduction techniques, alternative medicine and massage as a means to relieve stress and to learn to relax and experience a greater sense of health and well-being. At that time, Dr. Benson's ideas were considered near to scientific heresy. In 2000 his book was revised and reprinted, his views accepted as a necessary tool to relieve the level of stress we experience in daily life.

It is still surprising to know how many people have never had a massage and have no idea how to relax. Many people think they relax when sitting in front of the television. In most cases, watching television is hardly a relaxing experience! Have you ever observed people watching a sports event? How can one relax when watching the Olympics or an important horse race? Notice how viewers' bodies tighten and how they are yelling and cheering. Relaxed? Hardly! Even watching the news on television can be a stressful experience.

As with any learned skill, learning to relax while being touched takes practice. The more practice, the better the results. If you are being massaged by someone who talks a lot, you will find it more difficult to relax into the experience.

When beginning to massage your dog, realize that he needs practice to learn this new skill of relaxation through touch, just as we needed to relax in our first few massages. We need to teach him to relax to the differences in touch. One of the best ways to begin this teaching is by making the massage experience something different that is done away from other activity, such as you watching television or talking to another person at the same time.

First, set the environment. This creates a tone and a message that this is something different, something special from everyday interactions. When petting, we can be involved in other activities such as reading, watching television or talking to friends or family. The petting becomes and is part of the activity of the moment. When doing massage, turn off the television, put down your book and sit on the floor or on the couch so that your attention is solely focused on your dog.

Second, set the tone. Turn down the lights and put on soft music. If you like, light candles, especially when doing massage in the evening. Dogs respond to cues even better than we do. Just walk toward the closet where you keep dog treats for an immediate response cue! For massage, the music and softer lighting creates an environment that says, "We're doing something different now that is best received with focus and undivided attention." After several massages, your dog will know the cues and his nervous system will begin to relax and his attention will be on the massage. As you focus your attention, your dog will relax. Dogs learn and love the fact that massage is a special time where you both focus on the same activity.

Third, attitude is important for both teaching and learning. Your attitude while doing massage should be one of unconditional focus and giving. Enjoy the movements of your hands as you glide from stroke to stroke and focus on each bodily area, watching for any signals from your dog as he relaxes or as he feels pain. Use a quiet tone of voice and give much verbal assurance to your dog. All of this is part of the learning experience. If you raise your voice and make a command, you are changing the tone to something outside the intention of massage.

Also, consciously try to create consistent mood triggers for your dog as well as for yourself. Your voice tone is also a strong mood trigger. You want to elicit the relaxation response. What you say and how you say it will either elicit relaxation or some other response. You might try rubbing a relaxing scent on your hands or light some incense that isn't strong.

Once the mood is set, and you are relaxed, your dog will be relaxed and you can take time to explore and create new strokes and routines. In the beginning, you may need to find positions that work for your own comfort. Working with a dog often can mean sitting on the floor with him or being in new or uncomfortable positions. Dress in clothing that is not constricting such as sweat pants and t-shirts so that you can move comfortably and easily. When you move, and you will generally need to change position, do so slowly so the mood stays relaxed. With small dogs, sitting on the couch or on a chair is often easy to manage. With large dogs, sitting on the floor or on a small stool requires some getting used to in order to remain relaxed. After the first few massages, everyone settles into the relaxation of the experience.

❧ Notes ❧

Workbook Section

1. What helps you settle into receiving the most benefit from massage?

2. What was most difficult for you during your first massage?

3. What did your massage therapist do to help you relax?

4. List what you think would help your dog receive a massage.

5. List what you think would not help your dog receive a massage.

Chapter Three

Strokes — The Gift We Give Our Dogs

The one absolute, unselfish friend that man can have in this selfish world —
the one that never deserts him, the one that never proves ungrateful or treacherous — is his dog.
— George Graham Vest

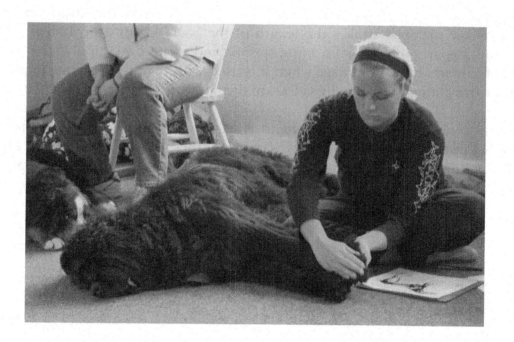

As previously mentioned, the massage stroke names as we know them today first appeared in the 1800s in European medical texts. For the most part, the same names are used today in training both human and canine massage therapists. For consistency, the names found in current massage texts will be used. After each description of a stroke, there will be an opportunity to practice it in the Workbook Section. Practice each stroke immediately after reading the description. By practicing the strokes, you perfect your style and gain the confidence you need.

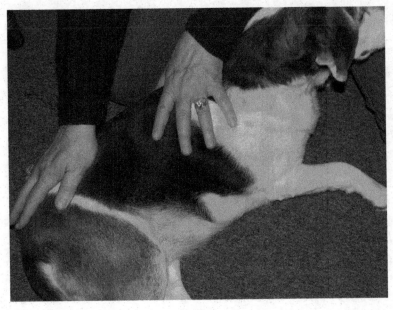

Effleurage: a gliding stroke. Effleurage is a French verb that means "to skim" or "to touch lightly." Effleurage is a stroke that is determined by pressure, speed, direction and rhythm. Effleurage is done horizontally along the length of the muscle or body part. It is the most frequently used stroke in massage and is used to begin massage after a resting position. Effleurage is a long, broad movement over an area of the body. It is done repeatedly while gradually increasing depth and pressure. This is the stroke experienced when a massage therapist strokes the length of the back, leg or arm. Effleurage warms the area and prepares the tissue for more specific and focused manipulations or strokes. Effleurage facilitates lymph drainage when it is used with light to moderate pressure with short, repetitive gliding from the digits toward the heart.

Effleurage is done by using the whole hand, fingertips or thumbs. Effleurage is also the stroke used to transition from one body part to another. When done quickly, effleurage strokes facilitate circulation and are very stimulating. When done slowly, effleurage is very soothing.

ᓂ Notes ᓂ

Workbook Section
Effleurage

1. Try doing several strokes down your dog's back by placing a hand on either side of his spine. Begin slowly so you feel the body part that is beneath your hands. The softness you feel is muscle tissue. Repeat the stroke several times using different parts of your hands. Describe what you feel.

2. Now try the same technique on your arm or leg. Begin at the wrist or the ankle and feel the muscle tissue beneath your hand. Notice where the bones are, and the shape of the muscles and body parts. Repeat this stroke several times. Each time use different pressure or even a different part of your hand. When doing these strokes you might want to use a bit of oil or lotion to provide more glide and less friction between your hand and your body part. How does this feel?

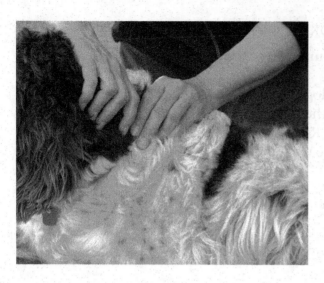

Petrissage: Petrissage also is a French word meaning "to knead." Petrissage or kneading requires the soft tissue to be lifted, rolled and squeezed. Instead of horizontal stroking, the focus is across the muscle or vertically.

Kneading or squeezing reduces muscle tension through its effect on the spindle cell proprioceptors in the belly or middle of the muscle. The action of kneading causes the muscle to feel less tense. Kneading actually tricks the muscle into relaxation because its action, whether squeezing or lifting, temporarily increases tension.

Kneading or petrissage mechanically softens the superficial fascia, the sheath that surrounds muscle tissue. When the fascia softens, space is created around the muscle fibers and the area becomes more pliable.

Kneading is a rhythmic motion that warms the muscle tissue and supports circulation and fluid exchange.

WORKBOOK SECTION
Petrissage

1. Try some kneading strokes on your dog's neck or back. Imagine you are kneading bread dough with the intention of making it more pliable. Try to make your motions rhythmic, smooth and flowing. Be gentle at first while your hands learn the technique. There will be plenty of time to go deeper once you feel comfortable with the stroke. Describe your experience.

2. Now try the same stroke on your neck. Apply a bit of oil or lotion to the area. This makes the stroke easier and much less painful. Remember, keep it simple, slow and rhythmic. Describe what you feel.

Skin Rolling: Skin rolling is a form of kneading that involves lifting the skin. Skin rolling has a very warming and softening effect on the superficial fascia. Although skin rolling can feel intense, the outcome is incredibly pleasurable and relaxing. Most dogs love skin rolling down the back on either side of the spine.

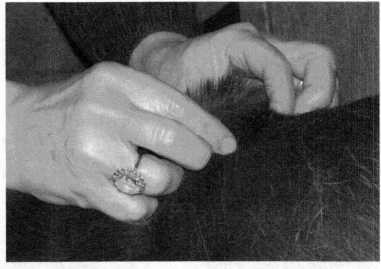

Skin rolling is also an excellent assessment tool. When doing skin rolling on your dog, the skin should roll easily under your fingertips. When you come across "stuck" skin, there may be an underlying problem that needs attention and a visit to your veterinarian.

To do skin rolling, lift a portion of the skin between your thumbs and first two fingers. Your thumbs become an anchor while your first two fingers "do the walking" by creeping forward. Pull more skin toward your thumbs as your thumbs roll slowly along the body part.

WORKBOOK SECTION
Skin Rolling

1. Begin at the base of the dog's neck with your hands next to each other. Lift a portion of skin between your fingers and thumbs. Begin to "walk" your fingers forward while your thumbs roll behind the lifted skin. The skin should lift easily. When it doesn't, you dog will let you know. Repeat this several times down the length of the back. What is your dog's response?

2. Try this on your thigh. You generally won't find the skin lifting as easily as it does on your dog and the sensation is a bit intense at first. Describe your experience.

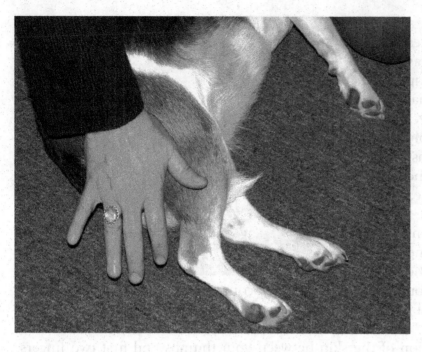

Compression: Compression is a movement that presses muscle tissue into the bony part beneath the muscle. It is the main method used in Shiatsu and other Asian bodywork practices. Compression is a downward motion into the soft tissue. The deeper the compression, the firmer the tissue is pressed against the underlying bone.

Compression can be done with the tips of the thumbs, fingertips, knuckles, palms and/or heels of the hands, fists, forearms and elbows. Whether you use thumbs or other body parts depends on the size of your dog as well as where you are applying the compression stroke. Compression in dogs is most often used in the hip area and hind limbs where the muscle mass is thicker and there may be more trigger points to be released.

Compression stimulates both the muscles and the nervous system. By compressing a muscle, you are passively causing the muscle fibers to contract. Although compression strokes are less desirable for a relaxing massage, the result is a combination of relaxation, release and alertness as the muscles being compressed probably have been holding tension.

Notes

WORKBOOK SECTION
Compression

1. Begin by putting your palm or heel of your hand into the thigh or hip of your dog. Go slowly at first to get a feel for the area and to notice how your dog responds to the compression. Press into the area with the heel or palm of your hand, stop and hold the compression while you take several long and slow deep breaths.

    As you relax, the muscle beneath your hand relaxes as well. Do one side of the hind end and then the other. Can you feel the muscle relax?

2. Practice on your thigh. No need to remove clothing or use oil here. When compressing into your thigh area, be sure you are compressing soft tissue or muscle and not just bony areas. Compressing into boney areas is quite uncomfortable. The key is to compress slowly and when you have gone as deeply as you can, stop and hold the compression for 4-6 slow breaths. This length of time allows for the brain to tell the muscle to relax. Describe the sensation of compression.

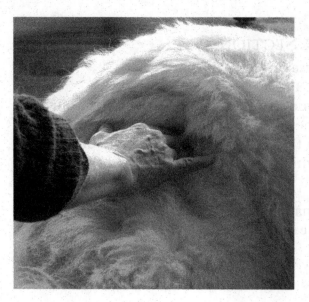

Vibration: Vibration is both a compression stroke and a trembling stroke. All vibrations begin with compression. Once you have compressed the muscle, the trembling action transmits the stroke to the surrounding tissue so that a broader area relaxes and lets go of tension. This stroke is used for short periods. The vibration movement is often done after compression strokes, especially if the muscle could use extra relaxation.

Vibration wakes up the muscle by stimulating nerve activity. The vibration confuses the muscle experience from its perception of pain to one of relaxation.

WORKBOOK SECTION
Vibration

1. Begin the vibration with a compression stroke into the thickest area of the dog's thigh or hip. Press in slowly and hold. While holding, let your hand begin to tremble. Release and try again on the other side. What was the dog's reaction?

2. Practice on your thigh by starting with a compression stroke. Hold briefly and then begin to let your hand tremble. Imagine that you are tricking the muscle into relaxation! How did this feel?

Shaking: Technically, shaking is a vibration stroke that works with muscle groups instead of one muscle. Shaking also uses confusion to cause the muscles to naturally relax. Shaking is a stroke that is used to warm and prepare the body for deeper work. Use your entire hand in a shaking motion. This is particularly effective when muscles seem tight and unready to release.

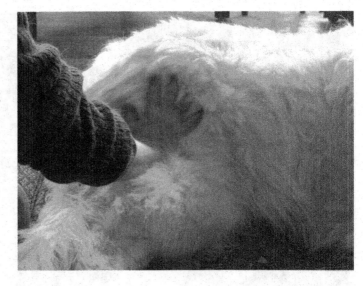

WORKBOOK SECTION
Shaking

1. Try the shaking stroke on your dog's thigh or shoulder. Try one side, then the other. Remember, shaking is used to warm an area for deeper work. Make it playful and light. How does your dog respond?

2. Shake the muscle that runs across the top of your shoulder. This muscle area is often tense on humans. Several minutes of shaking is often enough to release tension. How does this feel?

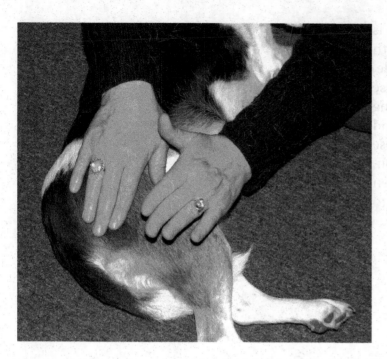

Tapotement (Percussion):
Tapoter is a French verb that means to rap, drum or pat. Tapotement is a springy motion that applies blows to the body at a rapid rate by using the sides or the palms of your hands in a cup position. Big dogs seem to enjoy this motion more than small dogs. Some dogs do not like this stroke as they find it jarring. Tapotement is a very stimulating stroke that enhances the sympathetic activity of the autonomic nervous system and is best done over large muscle groups such as thighs.

WORKBOOK SECTION
Tapotement (Percussion)

1. Try tapotement on your dog's thigh or shoulder. If your dog doesn't like it, he will let you know in no uncertain terms. How does your dog respond?

2. Try tapotement on your own thigh. How does it feel?

Friction: Friction is a series of small, deep movements within a local area, or short strokes that gradually move the length of a body part. Friction is generally done across the muscle fiber. Use your thumbs in alternating back and forth motions. Friction can prevent as well as break up local adhesions or scar tissue. Friction is never done on a fresh injury as these injuries need time to heal.

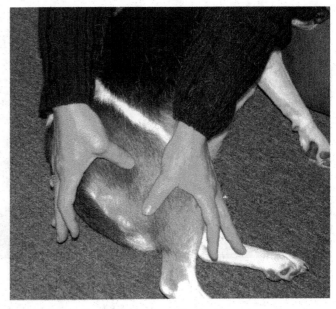

Friction reduces pain in an area by its warming action and by providing a counter irritation to an area. This creates a natural analgesic effect to the muscle area that results in relaxation.

In areas of the body where there are high concentrations of muscle tissue, as in the shoulders and thighs, friction helps keep the tissue soft and pliable. This is especially useful for active dogs such as those in agility training.

WORKBOOK SECTION
Friction

1. Alternate your thumbs in short movements on your dog's hip and thigh area. Begin gently and then go more deeply as your dog feels comfortable. Try again on the other hip or thigh. How does your dog respond?

2. Practice friction on your forearm below your elbow. These muscles become tense from daily activity. How does this feel?

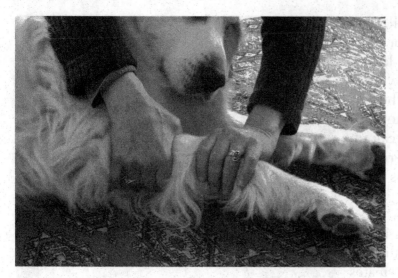

Wringing: A wringing stroke is done on the forelimbs or hind limbs. This two-handed motion resembles wringing out a wet towel. Use your full hands on a large dog, and your fingertips on a small dog. Begin at the top of the limb and wring your hands in an alternating motion as you work your way down the limb. Wringing is not a deep stroke; it is used for warming an area before deeper strokes are applied.

WORKBOOK SECTION
Wringing

1. Place your hands below your knee. Lightly begin wringing your hands from below your knee toward your ankle. Once the stroke feels comfortable, let your wringing motion be firmer so that you can feel the warmth being generated without feeling uncomfortable. How does this feel?

2. Now try this on your dog. Place your hands or fingertips at the top of the forelimb near the shoulder. Begin to lightly wring your hands from the upper forelimb toward the paw. This stroke may take several tries to feel comfortable. Once it does, let the wringing motion be firmer. Watch for signals from your dog to make certain that the stroke is not uncomfortable. How does your dog respond to this?

Rocking: Rocking is a soothing and rhythmic motion done with the intention of calming. It is a side-to-side and up-and-down movement, just like rocking a baby. This is a smooth and pleasurable movement, nothing abrupt, just a simple ebb and flow.

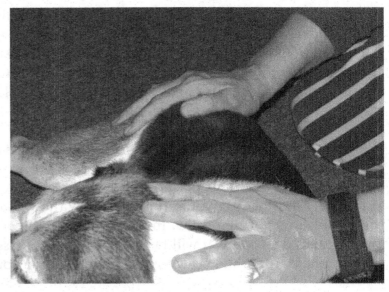

When rocking, use your full hand and begin slowly. Relax as you begin to do the rocking. The more you relax as the rocking motion begins, you and your dog will find a natural rhythm. Some rhythms are fast, others are slow and everyone has his own. You have to find what works for you.

Rocking is a great ending to a massage. Both doing the rocking as well as receiving it, allows us to settle into our inner rhythm of relaxation and deep calm.

WORKBOOK SECTION
Rocking

1. Place your hand on one side of your dog's hip and relax. Take a breath and let the rocking find the rhythm of the moment. There should be absolutely no effort to this stroke. How does your dog respond?

2. Place your hand on your abdomen and begin the rocking stroke. Take a breath and let the rocking lead you to a natural rhythm. The rocking spreads from the center up to the head and down to the toes. How does this feel?

These are the ten basic strokes. In addition, though technically not a stroke, is the laying on of hands. Laying on of hands is a calming, soothing and healing pause with the hands simply holding or resting on a body part. You may do laying on of hands over an injury, an arthritic joint, to calm an anxious dog, or to energetically end a massage session with a pause before lifting your hands away from the body. Laying on of hands is a quiet and natural part of many massage sessions.

From here you can begin to explore your own variations of these strokes that suit you and your dog. Practice them regularly so your hands get used to feeling the landscape of your dog's body. The more you practice these strokes, you will notice that certain ones seem to follow each other. Let yourself explore how the strokes fit together for you. Later, you will be able to put it all together in a routine that you can do regularly until your personal routine takes over and you will be doing your own massage. In the meantime, enjoy the practice, the learning and watching the bond between you and your dog grow!

↢ Notes ↣

Chapter Four

Canine Anatomy in a Nutshell

The head bone is connected to the tail bone.

— Anonymous

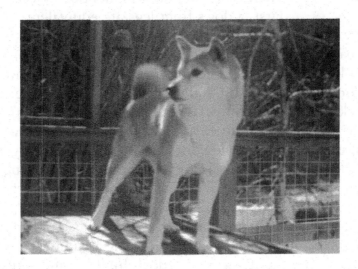

Anatomical Overview

Anatomy is an integral part of massage. Don't despair, we have made it quite simple.

For you, as your dog's caretaker, learning all the names of the muscles is not important. Understanding some basic information, however, is important when giving a proper massage to your dog.

Although canine professionals are extensively trained in anatomy, you know your dog well without scientific labels. Knowledge of basic anatomy allows you to offer a better massage to your canine companion and to detect early muscle and joint problems. In addition, understanding anatomy allows better communication with your veterinarian.

Human anatomy and human muscles, tendons and ligaments were studied long before dog anatomy. Therefore, many muscles in the dog are named after the human muscle counterparts. Interestingly, the muscle fibers in a dog go in the same direction as the dog's the hair/fur. This can be helpful when determining the stroke direction and the pressure of massage stroke.

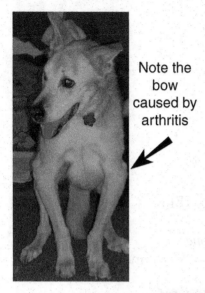

Note the bow caused by arthritis

In addition to learning anatomy, understanding conformation or the structure of your dog is important. Posture or stance of a dog may vary by breed and can play a role in creating muscle stress. These areas of stress can cause trigger points that become focal points for massage. Also, sometimes poor structure or a physical problem such as arthritis may cause slight or obvious stance variations. For example, the forelimb of a Labrador retriever is not shaped like a bulldog. However, an aging dog may have elbow bowing due to an arthritic condition. In this case, the forelimbs and neck would be a focus of massage.

There are a few points to mention before describing anatomy. First, a dog's front legs are equivalent to our arms with the noticeable difference that dogs use the front legs for weight bearing. The front legs are primarily used for balance and coordination and bear about 60% of a dog's weight. The exception is in short-legged dogs, such as Corgis or Basset hounds, who bear about 80% of their weight on the front legs. As a result of the increased weight on the forelimbs, problems can occur to the neck, shoulder, elbow, wrist or "finger" joints (digits). Veterinarians refer to these short-legged breeds as chondrodysplastic. The chondrodysplastic dogs originated as taller and more normally proportioned dogs but they had a dwarf gene. Breeders began breeding exclusively for the dwarf, or a shorter version of the taller dog. This also allowed for the ability to hunt animals that burrow or for nipping heels while herding!

Secondly, the rear legs are equivalent to our legs and are used primarily for propulsion forward. The rear legs bear 40% of the dog's weight. The anatomic components or parts of

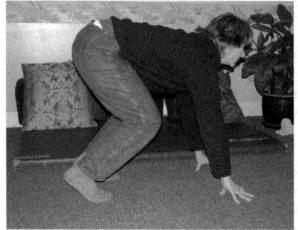

a dog's hind leg are similar to ours but have functional differences.

Consider the position of a dog that is standing on four legs. A dog's stance and motion is similar to a runner's position in a starting block. In visualizing a runner in a starting block, the arms are stabilized when rising onto the fingers and the legs rise up onto the toes. This position allows for the best propulsion from the starting block. The dog's stance is similar. However, the dog continues to walk and move in all gaits from this position. For the dog, this position gives the greatest propulsion from behind while allowing maximum balance and stability in the forelimbs.

Evolution has enabled dogs to move freely in this manner while people can neither move comfortably nor freely in this position.

Workbook Section

Do not do this if you have orthopedic or neurological problems.

1. Try getting into a runner's start position as shown above, so that you are on your fingers and toes. Be certain to hold your head up. Keep your buttocks lowered. Do you have more weight on your arms or legs?

2. How do your neck and lower back feel?

3. Now, try walking in this runner's position. What would happen if you were to try to lift both your arms off the floor?

4. Next, get into this runner's start position at the bottom of a staircase. Can you go up the stairs? If yes, describe your experience. If no, why not?

5. Now stand at the top of the stairs in the same position and think about a puppy, geriatric dog or vision-impaired dog walking down these stairs. Consider the problems he would have in trying to go down the stairs. **Do not try going down the stairs in this position.**

Properly trained a man can be a dog's best friend.
— Corey Ford

Overview: Head, Face, Ears and Neck

The head and face of a dog are in almost continual motion. The eyes widen, soften, stare and look side to side. The ears move when a dog is resting or tuning-in for distant or nearby sounds. The head cocks to one side in an expression of trying to understand new sights and sounds. The nose is constantly engaged because the dog smells and tracks the world around him. A dog's sense of smell is over 2 million times more acute than ours. They have 220 million olfactory cells to our 5 million. The lip may curl in a warning growl or be pleasantly relaxed.

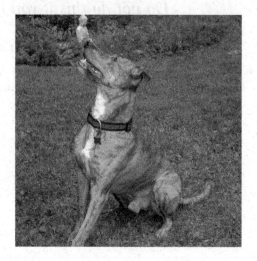

Simply stated, dogs carry a great deal of expression and tension in their faces. We believe that dogs bite to release great tension build-up. This can be seen in the dog that bites once and walks away as if nothing happened.

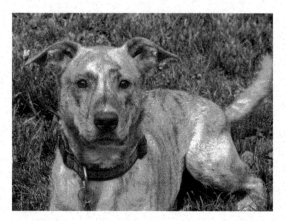

The Head and Face

While we think of the head and face as primarily skeletal, there are many underlying muscles in this area. These muscles are often overlooked in offering canine massage but are important components to full relaxation.

A relaxed dog enjoys having a massage start along the forehead and moving to the ear base followed by working toward the lips, mouth, face and chin. Be attentive to the large and small muscles of the face and lips and use a light touch that includes both small circles and long gentle strokes. Remember, stroking the nose toward the lip can cause the lip to curl. If this occurs, your dog is not growling as this is a normal neurological reflex.

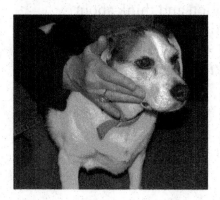

Anxious dogs may prefer having a massage begin at the neck or underneath the chin, followed by the ears, face and mouth once he is relaxed.

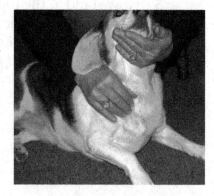

The Ears

There are many different ear types. See which ear type best typifies your dog.

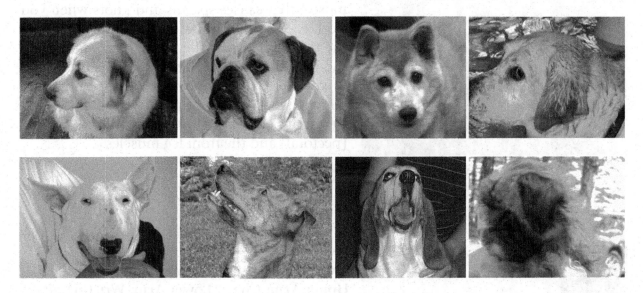

When massaging, always be attentive to any odors or tenderness near the ear. This can be a sign of infection and should be treated immediately by your veterinarian.

Ear stroking is one of the most relaxing and calming areas for massage on a dog. It is said that ear stroking can prevent shock associated with traumatic injuries and accidents. Begin with very small circles at the base of the ear, where the ear attaches to the head. Massage using circular strokes around the ear base. Then use long, light gentle strokes with your thumb and index finger going from the ear base to the tip. Feel the soft cartilage between your fingers and repeat this several times.

The Neck

The neck is comprised of many small and large muscles. The neck works constantly in helping to balance the head and body. The neck also adjusts the body balance during gait changes.

The neck flexes and extends when a dog is running, or in any movement. The neck bends fully when a dog bites or chews at any irritation on the ribs or on the tail.

When a dog is lame, the head will bob, rising for a forelimb injury and lowering for a hind limb injury.

The head and neck continually work against gravity, and adjust for balance. There is a large ligament in the neck that serves like a cable to help support the neck. This ligament is called the Nuchal ligament and attaches from the skull base to the shoulder blade area of the spine.

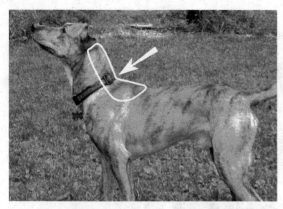

Trapezius. Arrow points
to area of "speed bumps."

The many large superficial muscles in the neck include the trapezius. In humans, this is the same muscle that causes spasms and knots when you work excessively on the computer. In your dog, the trapezius covers the entire neck area to the shoulder blades. If you feel across the neck base, this muscle feels like two little "speed bumps" lying parallel to each other. The neck muscles in the front begin to weave into the chest muscles (pectoral) and the front leg muscles.

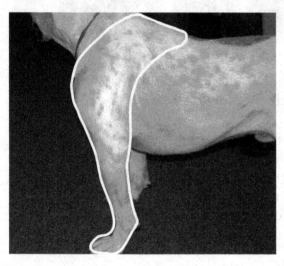

Forelimb, also called thoracic limb,
includes the areas from
scapula to paw tip.

Overview:
Front Legs/Forelimb, Scapula, Humerus, Upper Arm, Chest, Lower Arm, Wrist, Digits

The forelimbs are sometimes called thoracic limbs. The forelimb or thoracic limb includes all the areas from the shoulder blade (scapula) to the tip of the front paw. As previously mentioned, the front legs are anatomically similar to the human arm. However, due to the fact that dogs bear weight on their front legs, there are some noteworthy differences.

In general, the bones of a dog's front leg (arm) are proportionately smaller than in humans. The shoulder joint and clavicle (collar bone) is also much smaller in a dog. The clavicle is held together primarily by muscles and it has no bone to bone connection. This allows the neck, head and front legs to work together simultaneously with maximum power.

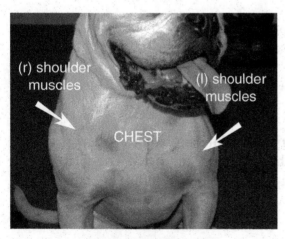

Chest muscles and
front view of shoulder muscles.

In terms of massage, the large shoulder and chest muscles do well with heavy, deep strokes while the finer muscles of the lower arm and paw do better with short, quick, light strokes due to the superficial nature of the muscles. Avoid massaging the bones of the shoulder blade (scapula) and lower leg, but massage the muscles overlying and surrounding these bones.

Workbook Section

1. With your dog lying down, lightly feel from his shoulder down his front leg. Where is the bone and where is the muscle?

2. Can you feel the difference between the large shoulder muscles and the fine muscles of the lower part of the limb?

Scapula or Shoulder Blade

The scapula also is known as the shoulder blade or, when you were a child, your grandmother may have called these "angel wings!" Those familiar with horses may know this area as the withers.

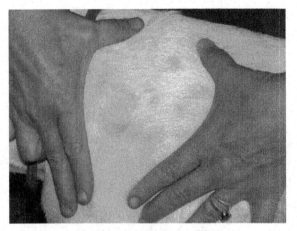

Hands are surrounding the area of the scapula.

The scapula has some mobility and a wide ridge in the middle called the "spine" of the scapula. The ridge (spine) in the middle separates and contains deeper muscles that help to move the front leg forward and back. The scapula and its deep muscles are covered by the large trapezius muscle, one of the large muscles that also extends into the neck. This muscle in both dogs and people is easy to feel because it lies immediately beneath the skin. Although the edges and margins of the scapula can be felt, the ridge (spine) of the scapula can not be felt due to the large trapezius muscle on top and the large muscles beneath. However, if muscles have gotten smaller (atrophy) the ridge will be protuberant.

The scapula margins that can be felt are on top, front and back. Do not massage the scapula bone. Instead, massage the muscle on top of the scapula and adjacent to these boney margins. Large muscle areas can be kneaded firmly, smaller circular or long strokes can be utilized at the margins outlining the scapula.

WORKBOOK SECTION
Scapula

1. While your dog is lying down, walk your fingers around the entire margin of the scapula to define the bone and muscle areas. Feel the top, front and back edges of the scapula. Note where the bone ends and the muscle begins.

2. Feel the heavy muscle over the middle of the scapula. Are there any knots or areas of tension? If so, describe.

3. Gently press down on the top, front and back edges of the scapula. Are you surprised at the amount of mobility in each of these areas?

The Humerus Bone

The upper arm bone is known as the humerus or humeral bone and many of the large muscles of the shoulder attach to this bone. The upper arm is also comprised of shoulder muscles that allow the forelimb to move forward and backward as well as some movement away from and toward the body. A dog has large, easy-to-feel muscles in the shoulder due to bearing weight on its front legs. The size of this muscle will vary based upon its breed. For example, a Newfoundland that originated as a carting dog will naturally have greater shoulder muscle than a Whippet that originated for high-speed running.

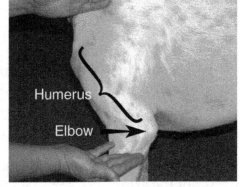

In this area, the muscles felt under the dog's skin include a portion of the trapezius, deltoid, biceps and triceps. The triceps are the muscle group at the back of your upper arm that becomes sore when doing repeated activity that requires holding your arm straight back in an extended position. In large shouldered, short-haired dogs, the triceps can feel very large. This is because there are four "heads" of muscle that create one muscle group.

There are many other deep muscles that lie beneath the superficial muscles. These can not be felt, but massage benefits all the muscle layers.

The large shoulder muscles can be relaxed with deeper and heavier strokes than might be applied to other muscle groups. Therefore, deep kneading, tapotement and long strokes are well tolerated and enjoyed.

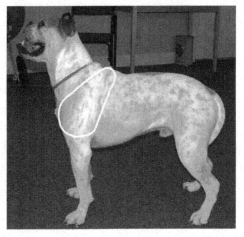

Area of large shoulder muscles.

The Chest

The muscles of the chest rest over the breast bone (sternum), on the under side of the dog, from the lower portion of the neck and down between the front legs. These large muscles include the pectoral muscles. A portion of these can be felt attached to the ribs and sternum.

The pectoral muscles keep the shoulders in line with the body during weight bearing. They extend and flex the shoulders and help to move the trunk of the body forward while the dog is in motion.

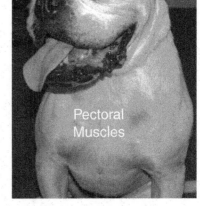

The pectoral muscles and entire chest are an area that dogs find relaxing and comforting when massaged. The large pectoral muscles do well with deep massage but gentle light strokes also are quite welcome!

Workbook Section
Humerus, Upper Arm and Chest

1. Feel the area of the upper arm on your dog. Can you feel the humerus bone?

2. How do the upper arm muscles differ in sight and feel from the lower portion of the arm?

3. Can you feel the junction where the humerus joins the scapula? Now move the leg gently forward and back. Can you feel the movement of the joint as the leg moves?

4. While the dog is standing and the forelimb is straight, gently and slowly move the forelimb from the shoulder, in all directions. Explore this and feel the shoulder as you move the leg. Are you surprised by the many directions the leg can move from the shoulder?

5. On the chest, what is the hair pattern and what direction does the hair lie/ grow? How is this different from the upper leg? What might this tell you about the direction of the muscle fibers?

Lower Arm (Antebrachium)

The two bones of the lower arm are the radius and ulna bones. At the bottom of the humerus, the top of the radial and ulna bones hinge together to form the elbow. Due to the required weight bearing and stability of the forelimbs, the dog's elbow differs from the human elbow. The dog elbow is more prominent as it allows for more muscle attachments. Since a dog carries 60% or more of its weight on the forelimbs, the elbow is more subject to arthritis and injury than in humans.

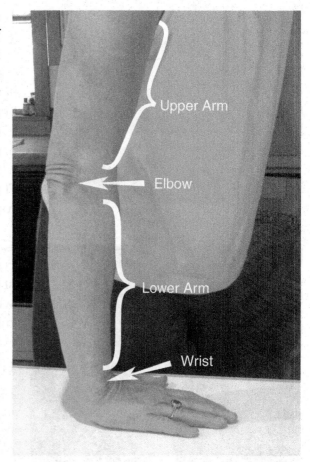

The radius is the main weight-bearing bone of the lower arm. For this reason, the radius has more distinct margins, which join it to the wrist bones, than occurs in humans. The ulna lies somewhat behind the radius and is thinner. The ulna is the longest bone in a dog's body.

There are many muscles that flex the forelimb and these are located primarily on the back portion of the lower arm adjacent to the ulna. The muscles that extend and rotate the lower arm are primarily located on the front of the lower arm adjacent to the radius.

The many muscles in the lower arm are smaller and finer than those in the shoulder and they do well with lighter effleurage massage strokes. Strokes in this area can be long or short but avoid discomfort by applying light pressure over any boney areas that lie under the muscle.

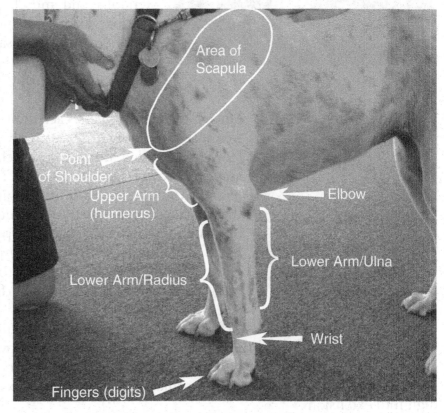

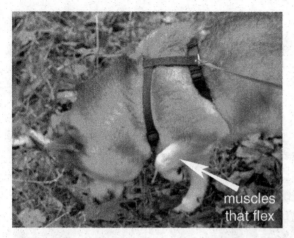

muscles that flex

Wrist (Carpus, Pastern)

The radius and ulna bones meet to form the bones of the wrist. This area in dogs is referred to as the carpus, carpal joint. Dogs have seven wrist bones while humans have eight. However, dogs have the same five carpal or hand bones as humans. A dog has a carpal accessory pad on the back side of the carpus (wrist). This pad helps to protect the wrist by absorbing concussive forces when jumping, running and making fast turns. The carpus (wrist) and carpal bones (hand) are covered with fine muscles to provide motion.

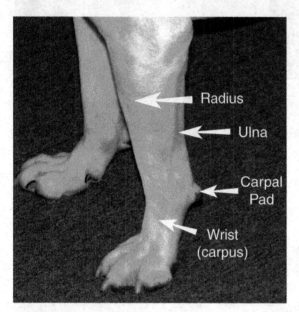

Radius

Ulna

Carpal Pad

Wrist (carpus)

Carpus massage must be light to avoid compression of the many underlying bones and structures. Gently rotate and extend the wrist while doing massage to allow relaxation of tired muscles.

Fingers (Digits)

Essentially, dogs walk on their fingers (digits) and this is sometimes referred to as digitgrade. As a result, dogs have more free floating bones called sesamoid bones. These bones allow the tendons and muscles to be pulled for quick flexion, extension and many sudden changes in direction. The sesamoid bones also reduce tendon and muscle stress at their digit insertions while weight bearing is occurring on the digits.

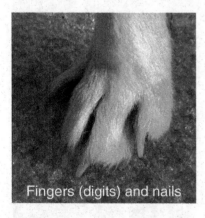

Fingers (digits) and nails

Much like human fingers, each digit has three joints. The digits we most commonly observe are the four located on the paw. However, the dog also has a dewclaw located on the inside aspect of the arm, near the carpus. This dewclaw is somewhat like our thumb, adding a fifth digit to the dog. The base of the dewclaw is connected to five muscles and tendons and is believed to support the wrist (carpus), hand (carpal bones) and fingers (digits) with quick turning. When the dewclaw is removed, some authorities believe this increases the incidence of carpal arthritis, especially in performance dogs.

If there is long hair between the paw pads, this should be carefully trimmed short prior to massage. The digits are covered with very small muscles that allow movement of the joints. Massage must be performed utilizing very gentle effleurage or circular pattern stroking. Move each of the finger joints in its normal range of motion, flex and then gently pull each digit into extension.

WORKBOOK SECTION
Lower Arm

1. Did you notice the direction of the hair pattern/growth on the lower arm? This pattern will help you in the direction of your massage strokes.

2. Gently feel your dog's elbow. Can you feel the bone in front (radius) and the bone in back that is slightly higher (ulna)?

3. Describe how is your elbow is different from your dog's?

4. Gently move the elbow forward and back while holding the elbow joint. Did you notice how this joint moves somewhat like a door hinge? Feel and notice the movement of the surrounding muscles as the joint moves.

Workbook Section
Wrist (Carpus)

1. Locate the carpal joint and gently explore the wrist (carpus) feeling the muscles and bones. Is there any swelling or tenderness?

2. Gently move the carpus to the right and left. Did you notice how it moves in these directions?

3. While the dog is lying on his side, lift the leg from the elbow. What happens to the wrist? Now lift your arm from the elbow. What happens to the wrist?

4. Can you find the carpal accessory pad (behind the carpus)?

WORKBOOK SECTION
Fingers (Digits)

Do not continue if your dog mouths you or growls when his paws are touched.

1. Feel each finger carefully exploring the bones, muscles and structure. How many joints can you feel? Flex and extend each joint.

2. How might excessive hair between the paw pads and fingers effect walking in snow? Running on slippery surfaces?

3. Does your dog have a dewclaw? If there is a dewclaw, move it gently. Can you feel how this is attached?

Overview: Spine, Ribs and Pelvis

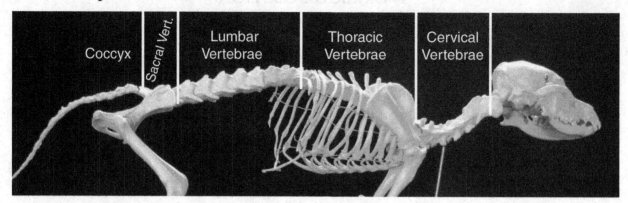

Coccyx | Sacral Vert. | Lumbar Vertebrae | Thoracic Vertebrae | Cervical Vertebrae

While we often think of the spine, ribs and pelvis as separate, this massive network of bones is contiguous and connected by many large and small muscles and ligaments.

The "backbone" that you feel is the vertebrae of the spine. You might think of this as a dotted line on a two-lane highway. The vertebrae are the dotted line and the muscles on either side are the lanes. The vertebrae in a dog project higher than the vertebrae in people.

As a dog ages or has a back problem, the muscles along the vertebrae atrophy or begin to shrink. The vertebrae (back bones) becomes more prominent and protrude. Also the vertebrae become thicker and less mobile. This is referred to as bridging. Warm moist heat or cold packs, padded by towels to protect the skin, can be applied to the back before massage. Your dog will let you know whether he prefers heat or cold! The spine of an underweight dog may also protrude and seem more pronounced than a normal weight dog.

The large cape muscles of the neck, previously described, protect the neck vertebrae (cervical vertebrae) making it difficult to feel bones at the top of the dog's neck. Some of the cervical bones can be gently felt on the underside of the neck. The large neck muscles on top of the neck tolerate deep massage work. In a dog with arthritis, the skin becomes "stuck" or tight as you move the skin over the spinal areas.

In consideration of the spine, do not massage on the bones (vertebrae) but massage the muscles. Light strokes, skin rolling and squeezing are excellent techniques for these muscles.

The spinal bones begin at the base of the skull and go into the pelvis. There are five components or parts of the spine: cervical (vertebrae start at head and go to the shoulder blade); thoracic (the ribs attach to the thoracic section, with the last rib attaching to the 13th thoracic vertebrae); lumbar (lower back area to the pelvic bone); sacral (lower part of the pelvis); coccygeal (bones of the tail).

As a point of interest, the spine of a dog differs from a human in that the vertebrae are taller but also there are a greater number of vertebrae. The numbering starts with the vertebrae closest to the head. Vertebrae are numbered for each of these sections. For example, the first cervical (C1) vertebrae is the one closest to the head and the seventh cervical (C7) vertebrae is at the area of the shoulder blades. The thoracic vertebrae follow C7 and begin with T1.

	Dogs	People
Cervical:	7 (C1-C7)	7
Thoracic:	13 (T1-T13)	12
Lumbar:	7 (L1-L7)	5
Sacral:	3 (S1-S3)	5
Coccygeal:	1 - 20	3
Total:	up to 50	26

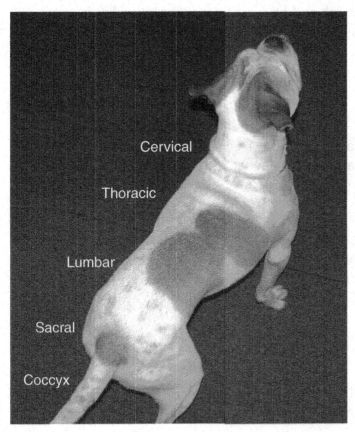

The reason dogs need more spinal vertebrae than humans is for increased flexibility with turning, running and jumping on four legs. In addition, humans have no tail so we only have three coccyx bones. The tail is important for balance, movement and serves like a rudder for a boat. Watch a dog's tail while jumping. The tail serves to adjust for turning and raises at the apex of the jump. Some authorities believe that tail docking can interfere with balance and make a dog more prone to injuries such as cruciate ligament tears to the knee.

There is one vertebra in the thoracic area at the area of thoracic ten (T10) that is lower than the others and can look like a dip or indentation. Do not be alarmed when you see this as it is normal and allows for lateral as well as up and down movement of the spine.

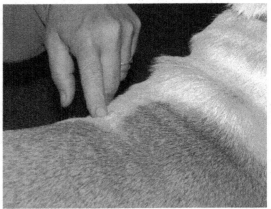

Thoracic T10 Dip

Workbook Section
Spine, Ribs and Pelvis

1. Beginning at the base of the head and top of the neck, feel the large wing-like bones that begin the cervical spine (C1). Are you surprised by the size of these bones?

2. Gently feel the under side of the neck and let your fingers explore what is muscle, what is bone and what is the soft tissue of the throat. How are each of these different?

3. Starting between the shoulder blades (scapula) feel for the vertebrae as you continue down the spine to the tail. Describe what you feel.

4. Feel each of the ribs starting at the spine and move toward the abdomen. Now count the ribs in this area (thoracic area). There are 13 ribs and these are usually easy to feel unless your dog is overweight. How many do you count?

5. Feel the area of the spine from where the last rib attaches to the area that begins the pelvis (lumbar area). Are there any knotted muscles in the adjacent areas?

6. Feel the entire area of the pelvis. Begin at the bones that feel like large bumps or wings and follow the pelvis to the tail base and slightly below. Can you visualize this area as a boney box for the sacral bones?

Overview: Hind Legs/Hind Limbs, Buttocks, Hip and Thigh, Knee, Lower Leg, Ankle

The hind limbs are sometimes referred to as pelvic limbs. This area includes the area of the pelvis to the tip of the hind paw. As previously mentioned, the hind limbs are similar to the human leg.

Buttocks

The buttock (gluteal) muscles rest on top of the pelvis. Imagine a runner in the starting block with the buttocks up. In this position, the buttock muscles appear to rest on top of the pelvis. The buttock muscles are proportionately smaller in dogs than humans. The gluteal muscles are responsible for extending the hip, allowing hip rotation in an inward direction and also permit some movement of the hind limb away from the body.

The buttock muscles often weaken and get smaller (atrophy) with hip problems such as CHD (canine hip dysplasia), hip arthritis or neurologic problems. In this case, rather than feeling healthy muscle with strong tone at the back portion of the pelvis, it will look or feel boney with poor muscle tone. This can be observed on one side or on both sides depending on the problem. It is easiest to see when looking at a standing dog from behind. This can also be seen in elderly dogs.

Hip and Thigh

The hip is a ball-and-socket joint and is surrounded by muscle. The pelvis creates a "roof" over the ball of the hip. The ball portion is the top of the large thigh bone (femur). The ball is held in place by ligaments, tendons and large muscles. The ball-and-socket nature of the hip allows movement in many directions — flexion, extension, inward and outward rotation, movement away and toward the body.

The ball of the hip attaches to the femur (large thigh bone) by a small neck of bone. The femur is the largest bone in the body and the large thigh muscles attach to various locations on the femur surface.

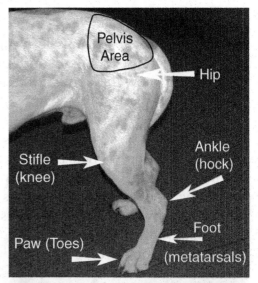

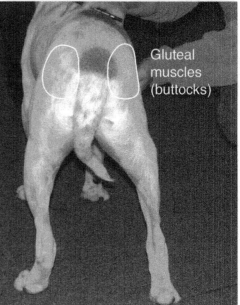

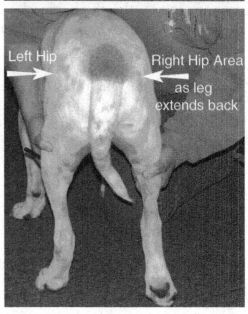

Thigh

Like humans, the major muscle groups of the thigh include the large quadricep muscles, a group of four muscles. These muscles help to extend the knee and one of these also flexes the hip. You know these muscles as those that burn climbing up hill or climbing stairs or using the stair master at the gym.

There is a band of muscle that rests in the front aspect of the thigh and it is called the sartorius. This muscle helps flex the hip and rotate the leg outward. The muscle is on top of the quadriceps muscles and often feels ropy or like a piece of inner tube. The sartorius muscle gets very tight when a dog is not capable of fully bearing weight on its hind leg. This is an up-and-down muscle and needs gentle massage with long strokes.

Compare the position of a human leg with dog in locating the quadriceps muscles.

Another large group of three muscles are the hamstrings that comprise the back portion of the thigh. These muscles primarily flex the knee, extend the hip and allow outward movement of the hip.

The thigh muscles, when viewed from the side and behind, should be equal on both legs. When there is injury to one of the hind-leg muscles, bones or primary joints, the thigh muscles on the injured leg often become smaller.

Deep kneading and percussion work well on the large thigh muscles. Note the hair pattern and follow this hair pattern when determining the direction of your strokes.

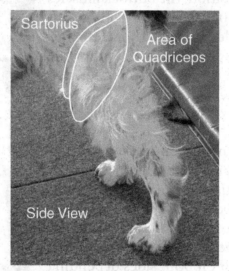

Sartorius

Area of Quadriceps

Side View

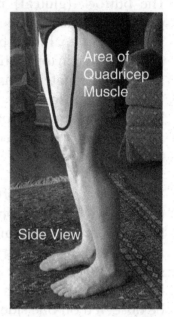

Area of Quadricep Muscle

Side View

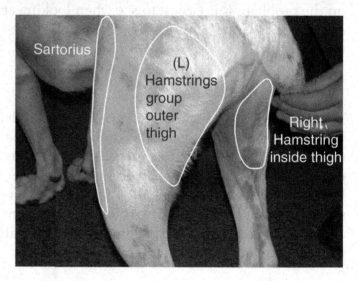

Sartorius

(L) Hamstrings group outer thigh

Right Hamstring inside thigh

Workbook Section
Buttocks, Hip and Thigh

1. While your dog is lying down, gently lift the hind leg 1-2 inches. Keep the leg parallel to the floor and gently rotated the hip in a circle, then flex it forward and backward. Does it move smoothly?

2. Look at your dog from behind while shifting the tail. Are both thighs equal in size? Look downward from the top of the buttocks muscles. Are both sides equal?

3. How do the thigh muscles differ from other muscles of the leg? Do the thigh muscles have stronger tone and larger size?

The Knee (Stifle)

The knee, also called stifle in a dog, is the joint that joins the femur (large thigh bone) with the large lower leg bone (tibia). The stifle joint is smaller, tighter and rides more forward in a dog than in a human. The joint flexes and extends much like a door hinge that allows a door to open and close.

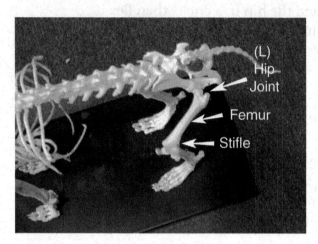
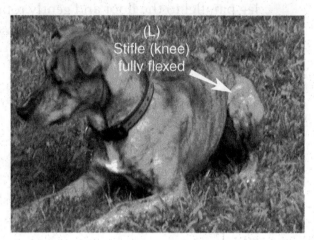

The ends of the femur and tibia that comprise the knee have a slick, smooth cartilage surface that allows the knee joint to move easily without pain. Inside the knee are two ligaments that create a cross and attach the femur to the tibia. One ligament keeps the lower leg bone (tibia) from slipping too far forward and is named the cranial cruciate ligament (CCL) in the dog or the anterior cruciate ligament in people (ACL). The other ligament keeps the tibia from slipping backward. This is the caudal cruciate ligament in a dog, or posterior cruciate ligament in people.

The knee cap (patella) is a floating bone that protects the knee joint. In people, the patella moves easily from side to side. In dogs, the kneecap is much smaller and feels like a hard pencil eraser. Unlike a human kneecap, it should not move but should fit tightly into a groove. The patella is held in place by a large tendon that originates off the quadriceps thigh muscles and attaches to the lower leg bone.

The knee cap (patella) is primarily a boney structure and should not be massaged. However, the muscles surrounding the knee, including the insertion of the thigh muscles on the front and back, lend well to deep massage. The soft tissues around the knee on either side also can take a light massage that dogs find enjoyable. Dogs that have had a previous knee injury or have knee arthritis will have a bump on the inside of the knee and that knee may feel slightly larger than the other knee. Remember to massage lightly over any boney areas of the knee.

WORKBOOK SECTION
Knee (Stifle)

1. With your leg held straight and relaxed, move your knee cap gently from side to side. How much does your knee cap move?

2. Try to feel your dog's knee cap. Follow the muscle in front of the thigh downward to the first small bump you feel. This is the knee cap. Feel its size compared to yours. Did you notice the lack of movement from side to side?

3. Move the lower portion of the leg forward and back while holding the knee in place. Did you notice the amount of flexion and extension of the knee?

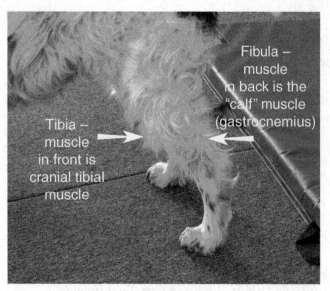

The Lower Leg

The lower leg is primarily made up of two bones—the tibia and the fibula. The tibia is the larger of the two bones and is located in the front portion of the lower leg. The tibia is the weight-bearing bone of the lower leg. The fibula sits behind the tibia and does not bear weight in a dog but serves as a primary bone for muscle attachments at the back of the lower leg.

There are several muscles in front and on either side of the tibia, one of the largest is named the cranial tibial muscle and helps to flex the hock (ankle). One of the major muscles in the back of the lower leg is what is commonly referred to as the calf muscle or gastrocnemius that flexes the knee and extends the hock (ankle).

WORKBOOK SECTION
Lower Leg

1. Beginning beneath the knee to the area of the ankle, feel the front aspect of the lower leg. Can you feel the tibia (bone) and the adjacent muscles?

2. Beginning behind the knee to the area of the ankle bone, feel the back of the lower leg. Can you feel the calf muscle (gastrocnemius)?

3. Can you feel the Achilles tendon that extends from the base of the calf muscle to the ankle bone?

Ankle (Hock)

The tibia and fibula (lower leg bones) join the bones of the feet at the ankle joint known as the hock in a dog. Remember, unlike humans, a dog's weight bearing is on his toes and not his foot. Hence, the back portion of the ankle is the heel bone. The Achilles tendon attaches from the heel to the calf muscle allowing the ankle to flex and extend.

The ankle and foot are comprised of many bones and many small muscles that connect these bones. Take the time to massage the small muscles of the ankle, feet and paws with gentle massage strokes.

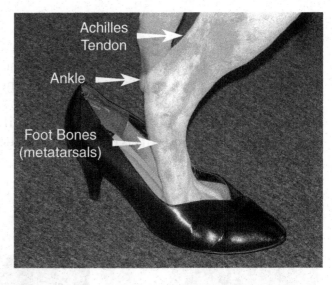

WORKBOOK SECTION
Ankle (Hock)

1. Feel the area of the ankle joint. Gently move the ankle forward (flex) and now straighten (extend). Does this move smoothly? What happens to the Achilles when you move the ankle? Can you feel it shorten and lengthen?

2. How is your ankle different from your dog's ankle?

Foot (Metatarsals)

The terms "foot" and "paw" are sometimes used interchangeably and can cause confusion to dog owners. Also, these terms are sometimes used to describe the front limb and the hind limb. Correctly speaking, the "foot" should be referred to when discussing the metatarsal bones of the hind limb. These bones, much like in humans, extend from the ankle (hock) joint to the toes. One obvious difference is that humans walk on their foot bones (metatarsals) and this is called plantigrade. Dogs walk on their toes and this is called digitgrade.

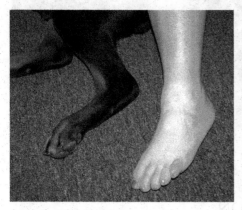 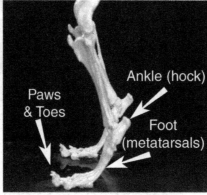

Ankle (hock)

Paws & Toes

Foot (metatarsals)

The paw begins at the distal portion of the foot bones and includes all aspects of the toes and pads, muscle and bone. We think of the metatarsals as mostly bone, but there are many small and important muscles, tendons and ligaments in this area. Due to the superficial nature of the foot bones, the muscles of this area are best massaged lightly with sweeping strokes that begin at the ankle and extend off the toes. Wringing and gentle friction rub are also useful strokes in this area. Remember to massage the front and back aspects of the feet.

Workbook Section
Foot (Metatarsals)

1. Feel the long bones of the foot on the front and back aspects. Can you feel how these bones join to the ankle and the toes? Can you differentiate between the muscle and the bone?

2. Observe how you walk on your foot (plantigrade) and your dog walks on his toes (digitgrade). Can you see the difference?

Overview: Toes (Hind Digits), Paws and Nails

Toes

Each of the toes begins at the bottom of the metatarsal bones and ends at the nail. There are four toes plus a dewclaw on each hind limb. Some experts believe that the hind dewclaws are functional and should not be removed. Breeds such as the Great Pyrenees and Briard have double (or more) dewclaws. These double dewclaws are boney looking rather than appearing like a nail.

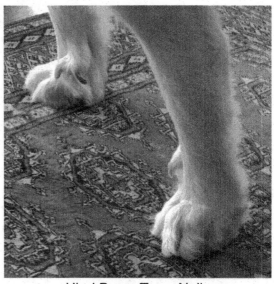

Hind Paws, Toes, Nails

The toe has three distinct joints that flex and extend and are covered with small muscles and tendons that work like pulleys. The toes and nails are used for gripping ground as a dog moves forward, backward, or changes directions from side to side. Therefore, in working and aging dogs the toes are prone to arthritis and are often over looked.

Paws

The pads of the hind paw have one large pad at the back of the paw called the metatarsal pad. The other smaller pads are called the digit pads. Pads are prone to injury from use on abrasive surfaces (snow, concrete, rocks, etc.) and can become dry or crack. The pads are important in cushioning the toe bones and should be monitored.

Remove all hair between the pads. Long hair serves like slippery socks and can cause falls, especially in senior dogs! Snow, burrs or twigs can become lodged in the hair and cause limping. Apply oils and massage the pads regularly unless your dog does not like his feet rubbed. Massage using soft circular strokes and be certain to carefully stretch each of the toe joints.

Nails

The nail or claw grows from its base at an average rate of 2 mm per week. Nails that are not worn down naturally must be trimmed frequently or nail length interferes with ambulation. Normally, nails should be trimmed at least monthly to provide proper paw health. If untrimmed, the nail can become imbedded in the paw and cause infection and lameness. Any alteration in proper movement can cause muscle knots, aches and joint strain. Use the massage time to check the length of the nails. If the nails are long and need cutting do NOT do this during your massage; wait for a more appropriate time. Most dogs do not like their nails trimmed and they may begin to associate a calming massage with a stressful nail-cutting event.

Workbook section
Toes, Paws and Nails

1. Feel each toe and the joint of each toe. Move each of the three joins separately on each toe. Are you surprised that the toes are so flexible?

2. What is the condition of your dog's nails? Is the nail wear equal on each toe? What might differing nail wear suggest to you?

3. Is there a dewclaw on each hind foot? Some breeds may have more than one!

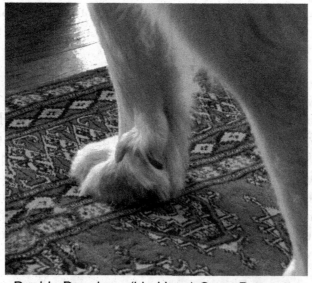

Double Dewclaws (hind legs) Great Pyrenees

Chapter Five

Stretches

A dog is the only thing on earth that loves you more than he loves himself.
— Josh Billings

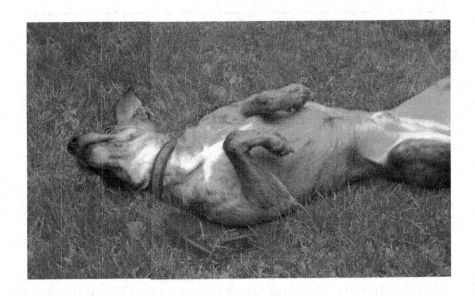

Gentle joint stretching is woven and integrated throughout the massage experience. Stretching assists in healthy joint mobility and joint integrity as well as keeping the muscle fibers toned. Repetitive motion with no stretching leaves joints and muscles stiff. We recommend that gentle stretching be included while massaging your dog.

Dogs automatically stretch to reduce muscle tension and to maintain joint flexibility. Most common are the cat-like back arch and the play bow position when a dog arises from a nap, or descending from a height. Large dogs can be seen stretching with full extension of the back and hind limbs. They place their front legs on the ground leaving their hind legs back, and small dogs do the same by extending their front legs and arching their back into a similar stretch. The head often looks up to the ceiling as the back is fully extended. The stretches are similar to the downward dog, the cat stretch and the beginning phase of the cobra that many are familiar with in yoga practice or stretching classes.

Canine stretching can reduce risk of muscle injury, increase relaxation and improve body awareness. Stretching also improves muscle and joint flexibility because muscle fibers are lengthened. The benefits of stretching include increasing blood flow to muscles involved with joint motion. This increases muscle fiber tone and reduces muscle tension. The improved elasticity and pliability of muscle, tendons, and ligaments permits faster and freer motion with less risk of injury.

Additional benefits include improved stride length and active range of motion. While loosening joint adhesions (scar tissue) and muscle spasms, stretching also improves coordination. In addition, there is improved perception regarding limb movement through space, known as our sense of proprioception. This is especially helpful for neurologically impaired dogs.

KEY POINTS TO REMEMBER WHEN STRETCHING

1. Consult your veterinarian if you notice stiff, restricted swollen or warm joints or if you are at all unsure of your dog's health.

2. Never over stretch a joint. It is always better to under stretch than overstretch.

3. Massage the muscles before stretching the joint. This assures that the muscles are warm, relaxed and there is adequate circulation to the area.

4. Hold the stretch steady and take a deep breath. Do not bounce or pulsate the joint. Hold each stretch for 15-20 seconds until you feel mild muscle relaxation.

5. Stretch the joint until there is slight resistance and then STOP. Do not stretch past this resistance.

6. Stiff joints can be loosened with warm packs prior to stretching.

7. End the stretch with long slow strokes down the limb as you approach the next massage area.

Getting Started with Stretching

Begin with general, relaxing massage moving with the muscles surrounding the joint. The stretch must be part of the massage flow, not a separate component. Think about the normal movement of your dog before applying the stretch. The limb should be guided according to the dog's natural movement.

During a relaxing massage with stretching, your dog should be lying down in a comfortable position if at all possible. Do *not* twist or apply torque to the joint. Carefully follow the pictures and descriptions in this chapter for each sequence of stretching.

Some joints may have restrictions due to previous injury, misuse, lack of use, aging or even surgery. Never be in a hurry to correct these restrictions. Restrictions will slowly release with daily stretching and working in conjunction with your veterinarian and therapist's recommendations. Be tender, gentle and patient. Over stretching can tear muscle, tendon or ligament fibers. Each stretch is performed with consideration of joint flexibility, tolerance and muscle tension. Once the stretch is completed, return the limb to the neutral or normal position.

The following photos, with descriptions of the stretches, will help build your skill level. Keep in mind, there are many more stretches. However, these are the basic stretching movements that can be used to keep your dog's joints healthy and flow well with massage strokes.

Forelimb Stretching

Elbow Flexion — "Flies off the ears" or "a salute"

Gently press near the elbow with one hand. Bring the lower portion of the forelimb up to the ear. The paw is placed on top of the ear while the limb is maintained close to the body. This exercise maximally flexes the elbow. Return to a straight neutral position.

Shoulder Extension or "forward stretch"

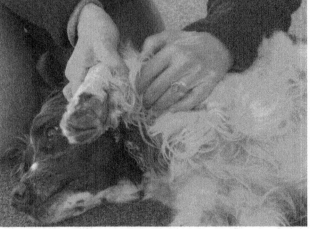

Elbow Flexion

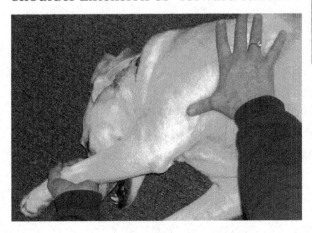

Forward Stretch

Extend forelimb toward the dog's nose. This is performed by gently holding the wrist (carpus) and lightly pressing the elbow forward. The exercise extends the shoulder, carpus and elbow. Normally, the forelimb should move easily forward to nose/eye level. Return to neutral position.

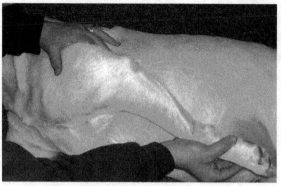

Shoulder Flexion or "backward stretch"

The forelimb is gently pulled back toward the hind leg. This is performed by gently holding the carpus as the shoulder glides back. Once the shoulder is flexed, the elbow can slowly be straightened. The exercise flexes the shoulder and extends the elbow. Normally, the forelimb should flex and the elbow should easily straighten. Return to neutral position.

Backward Stretch

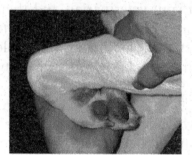

Wrist Flexion or "wrist (carpus) stretch back"

The paw pad is flexed to lie flat on the back (posterior or caudal) aspect of the forelimb. The exercise maximally flexes the wrist/carpus. Normally, the paw pad will move without resistance to touch the back of the forelimb. Return to neutral position.

Wrist Flexion

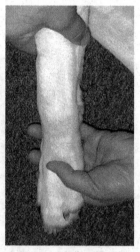

Wrist (carpus) Extension

The wrist (carpus) is fully straightened (extended) by placing one hand immediately above the wrist joint and using your other hand to straighten the "hand" and paw. Normally this should create a completely straight line along the lower arm to the paw. The wrist may not fully extend if wrist arthritis is present.

Wrist Extension

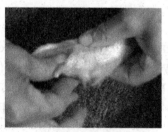

Finger "Digit" Flexion and Extension

Support the "hand" and paw and gently bend (flex) then straighten (extend) each of the finger (digit) joints.

Digit Flexion
and Extension

Hind Limb Stretching

Hip Rotation

Rotate the hip five times in each direction while holding the thigh at the knee (stifle) or slightly higher. *The leg should be parallel to the other hind limb.* Normally the hip joint should move freely.

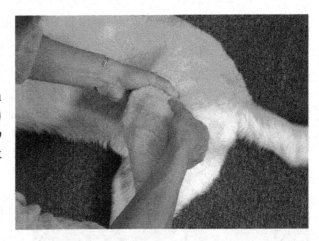

Hip Extension or "Puppy Stretch"

Stretch the hip gently moving back the entire leg while holding the ankle (hock) area. Simultaneously use downward stroking at the front (anterior or cranial) aspect of the thigh. Think of how far a puppy will stretch the leg out behind himself. Keep in mind that older dogs will not stretch as far as a puppy. Normally the hip extends fully but can be restricted if there is arthritis or hip dysplasia.

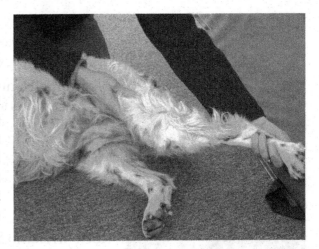

Hip Abduction or "Fire Hydrant Move"

Gently lift the thigh (abduction) to expose part of the abdomen and groin. Think of how high a male dog lifts its leg to urinate on a fire hydrant. Once the leg is abducted, gently rub the crease of the groin with special focus on the forward third of the groin crease. The exercise helps to loosen the hips and increase flexibility of hip muscles.

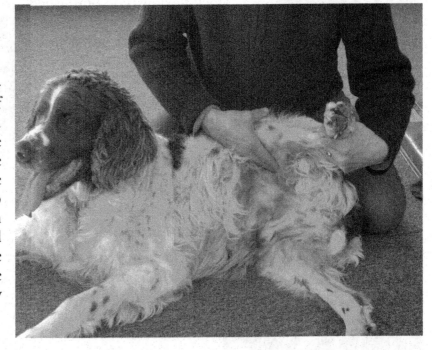

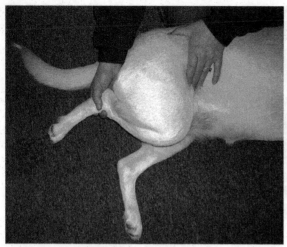

Knee (stifle) Stretching

Knee (stifle) Flexion

Flex the stifle by gently placing the heel bone (hock) onto the seat bone (ischial tuberosity of the pelvis). Normally, this maximally flexes the knee. However, restriction can occur with arthritis in the knee or immediately following knee surgery (cruciate ligament repair of luxating patella).

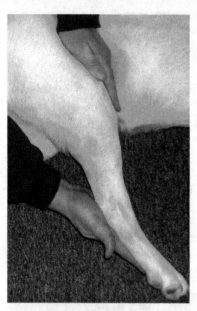

Knee (Stifle) Extension

Extend the stifle by gently holding the hock and gliding the leg toward the front limb. At the same time, gently press on the top of the anterior (front) thigh to straighten the stifle (knee) joint. The goal is to get the stifle joint as straight as possible. The exercise maximally extends the knee and is often times initially restricted after knee surgery.

Hock Stretching

Hock Flexion

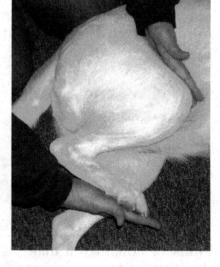

Hock flexion is accomplished by moving the top of the paw pad up toward the knee (stifle). The thigh often has to be pressed gently in a downward direction or the limb will rise away from the compression. Normally, the top of the paw will come within 1½ to 2 inches of the stifle. Hock flexion is compromised with any knee or hock problems. The exercise allows for maximal hock flexion.

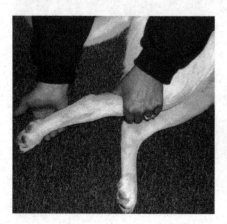

Hock Extension

Hock extension is accomplished by holding the leg joint above the paw on the front aspect of the leg just below the knee. Then straighten the "foot" and paw. Normally, the hock should straighten easily.

Toe (Digit) Stretching

Support the foot and paw and gently bend (flex) and straighten (extend) each of the digit joints.

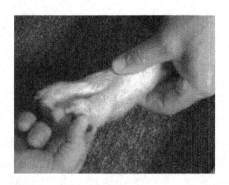

Tail Stretches

Dogs laugh, but they laugh with their tails.
— Max Eastman

The tail is a series of bones and joints. As you will recall in Chapter 4, Canine Anatomy, the vertebrae of the tail are known as the coccygeal or caudal vertebrae. The number of joints depends on tail length. Some dogs have more than 20 joints and vertebrae in their tails. The purpose of tail stretching is to relax the base of the tail and lower back by straightening the spine.

Most dogs love the tail stretches because they find it relaxing and they cannot do these stretches by themselves. Be certain to watch your dog's body language and facial expression. Keep in mind that some dogs do not like their tails touched and need time to get used to these stretches.

Tail Pull

Begin by gently squeezing each bone in the tail. Be especially gentle at the tail tip. Once this is completed, place one hand on the tail base and softly grasp the tail approximately two inches from the tail base. Gently but firmly pull the tail directly away from the tail base. This applies gentle traction. Hold the tail stretch for about ten seconds, then slowly over another ten seconds release the tail. Repeat this five times. **Never jerk the tail and do not grasp the tail too tightly.**

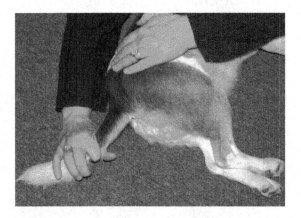

Tail Circles

Gently place one hand at the base of the tail and carefully press the tail toward the body.

This creates a rounding curve of the tail and relaxes the tail base. Rotate the tail in a circle clockwise and counter clockwise for 3-5 rotations in each direction.

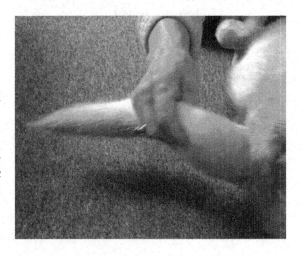

WORKBOOK SECTION
Forelimb, Hind Limb and Tail Stretches

1. Think about how each limb and joint moves in a play bow, ear scratch and bone holding. Describe what the limbs and joints look like. For example, the forelimb moves back and forth in a walk, extends with a play bow, ear scratch and bone holding. The hind limb runs, lifts a leg, and extends back to stretch. The head looks up at a squirrel in a tree, and down to food on the ground, cocks side to side at odd sounds, and moves to bite an itch. The tail (even with short-tailed dogs) holds high, low and wags back and forth. How many more moves can you list or describe?

2. Move each limb and joint as described in the stretching chapter. Do you notice any restrictions?

3. Describe your dog's tail.

4. Notice how your dog uses his tail when:

. . . . greeting other dogs

. . . .when he is happy

. . . .when he is sad

. . . .when running

. . . .when jumping

Chapter Six

A Massage Routine

The dog has the soul of a philosopher.

— Plato

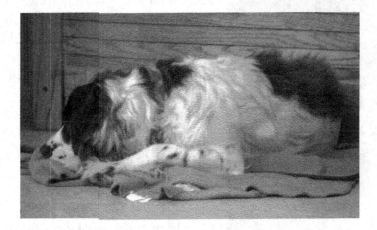

It is now time to pull it all together and do a massage. Before beginning, keep in mind the key points that we have emphasized throughout the book. Some of these key points are worth reviewing here.

Avoid massaging boney areas such as joints and the spine. Massage is focused on the soft tissue or muscles of the body. Massaging bone hurts. Massaging soft tissue is enjoyable and relaxing.

Set the Tone

Begin the massage on your dog by finding a comfortable position for both of you. Become aware of your breath. Now, softly, deepen the breath into your belly, allowing each breath to relax you. Breathe in this manner for several deep breaths while you begin to connect with your dog's body, mind and spirit.

Remember to "speak" softly with words or thoughts to your dog throughout the massage. This lets him know this is his special time. Though the touch is different in focus and intention, it is soothing and relaxing. Watch as your dog relaxes with each stroke and movement.

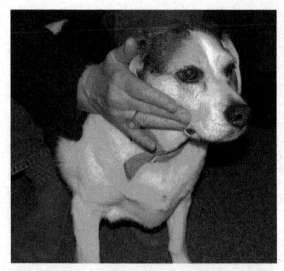

The Massage

Start the massage contact by placing your hands on an area with which your dog is comfortable. This area may be along the neck, the shoulder, the top of the head or back. Take a few moments stroking this area. Then work toward the top of the neck. Use long slow sweeping strokes from the neck and along the back to the tail base. Repeat this stroke at least three times. Notice what you are feeling beneath your fingers and hands.

Notice any areas of tension in your dog. Begin by massaging the entire face. Using your thumbs on either side of the nose, initiate long soft strokes and/or small gentle circles along the muzzle moving slowly from the nose toward the eyes and ears. Follow the hair pattern of the face. Alternate your thumb strokes, massage around the eyes and forehead. Begin to feel your dog relax.

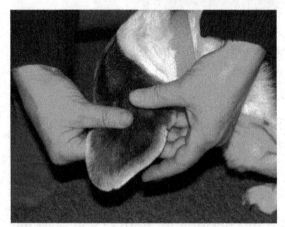

Move toward the base of the ears and use gentle circles around the base. Like the muzzle, the ear base holds a great deal of tension and needs attention. Massage the front edge of the ears from the base to the tip.

Gently pull the ear from the base toward the tip, stretching the ear slightly backwards. Rub the tip of the ear between your fingers. Notice all that your fingertips feel.

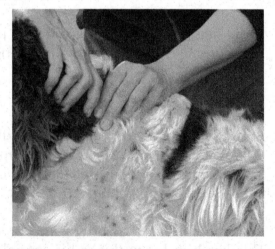

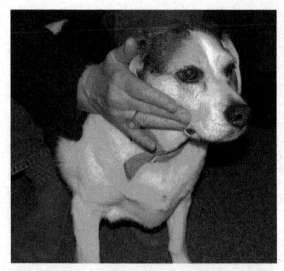

Massage one side of the neck for large dogs and both sides of the neck simultaneously for small dogs. Let your hands explore the muscles of the entire neck and shoulder. Massage the crest of the neck by lightly squeezing the muscles. Increase the pressure slightly with both hands along the entire upper neck from the base of the skull to the shoulders. Think about the texture and quality of the muscle you are feeling and note the location of the bone and muscle. Also note if the muscles feel soft and easy to move.

From the area of the neck, move slowly toward the shoulder. Use long strokes as you move from the neck to the shoulder. Begin with light strokes and slowly increase pressure over the shoulder with circles and kneading. This is a large muscular area and responds well to deeper pressure than other areas of the body.

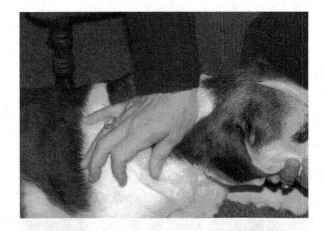

Work toward the front chest area using similar strokes over the chest muscles. Lighten your pressure over the breast bone (sternum).

Use long slow strokes as you move from the shoulder area toward the elbow and lower front leg. Sweep these downward strokes from the shoulder to the front paw. Avoid the paw itself if your dog is sensitive about paw touching. VERY soft thumb strokes or very gentle circles can be used in the muscle areas near the elbow. If your dog has elbow arthritis use a laying on of hands at the elbow area and work the area above and below the joint.

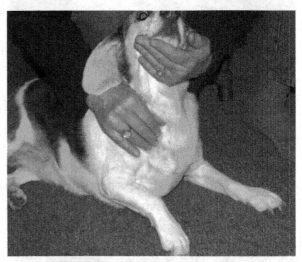

Continue down the limb using a combination of quick thumb strokes, gentle muscle squeezing and wringing. Repeat each leg stroke 3-4 times.

If your dog accepts paw massage, use long soft strokes on the top portion of the paw. Each paw pad can be tenderly squeezed and each toe can be gently pulled and massaged.

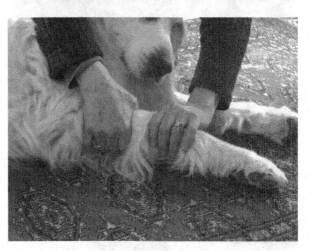

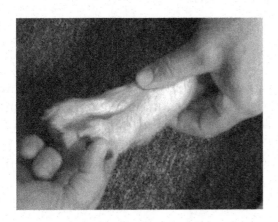

Forelimb Stretching with Massage

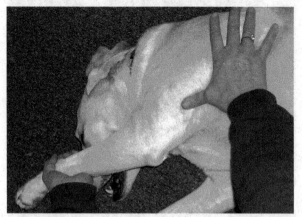

Shoulder Stretch

Now that the entire forelimb and neck is relaxed, you can begin to stretch the foreleg forward into a long stretch. As soon as you feel ANY resistance, STOP. While holding the stretch for 15-20 seconds, massage the muscle areas above and behind the elbow. If your dog pulls away at any point, *immediately* release the stretch. When the stretch is complete, carefully bring the limb back to neutral position.

Now, go to the front of the lower forelimb. Slowly move the limb backward toward the hind leg. This helps to stretch the front of the chest. As soon as you feel ANY resistance, STOP. While you hold the stretch for 15-20 seconds, massage the chest muscles (pectorals) as well as the muscles in the upper front portion of the forelimb. Once the stretch is completed, return the limb to neutral position and apply long strokes to the limb.

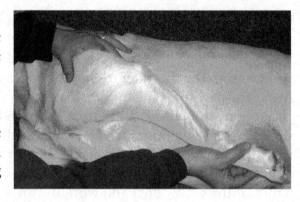

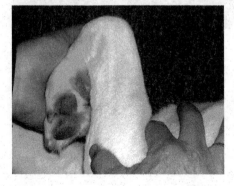

Elbow Stretch

Next, gently bend the forelimb at the elbow and move the wrist (carpus) toward the chin to the ear. As soon as you feel resistance, STOP. Hold the stretch for 15-20 seconds. If possible, with the free hand, continue to massage the muscles being stretched. Once the stretch is completed, return the limb to neutral position and apply long strokes to the limb.

Wrist (carpus) Stretch

Use a long stroke and move to the wrist area. Gently, bend the paw at the wrist toward the underside of the forelimb. The motion is one of folding and bending. When you feel resistance, STOP. While holding the stretch for 15-20 seconds, massage the underside of the lower forelimb. Return the limb to neutral position.

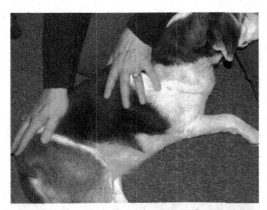

Start at the Back

Repeat several long strokes from the shoulder, down the forelimb toward the paw then return to the upper back. Now initiate several long but firm strokes along both sides of the back from the neck to the tail.

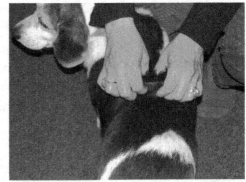

Beginning at the shoulders with a hand on either side of the spine, do some skin rolling down the entire back to the tail. Roll the skin between your fingers and thumbs, pulling the skin up with your fingers and gliding forward with your thumbs. Your fingers are doing the walking with your thumbs sliding behind. This stroke is fun to do and your dog will LOVE it!!

With your hands on either side of the spine, create small circles with your finger tips, working along the back toward the tail. Avoid the boney area of the spine.

Follow the spine to the pelvic bones and the sacrum. Tenderly vibrate the sacral area with your fingertips for 15-20 seconds. Finish on the sacrum with several clockwise and counter-clockwise circles using your fingertips for light strokes or thumbs for deep strokes. For larger dogs, use your full palm.

Massage the muscle area surrounding the hip using soft circular motions. Move from the hip to the thigh and upper leg areas. At the thigh, use deep circular strokes and compression, using your palm for deep pressure into these large hind-limb muscles.

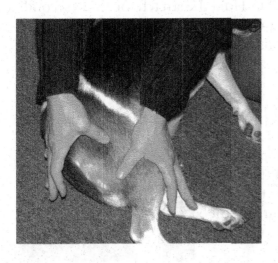

Now, move your strokes to the back of the thigh. Here you find hamstring muscles. Use long sweeping strokes from the pelvis toward the lower leg. Include the muscles of the back of the inner thigh. Quick thumb strokes, in both downward and outward motions, are also relaxing. Pay special attention to any areas where there seems to be bunching or thickening of the muscle.

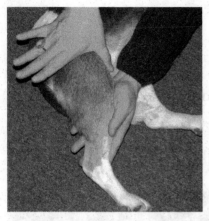

Use long strokes to move to the area below the knee (stifle) toward the ankle (hock). Include both the front and the back of the lower hind leg. Continue to massage the lower portion of the leg with squeezing, wringing. Now move to the hind foot and paw. Massage the paw and toes.

Hind Limb Stretching with Massage

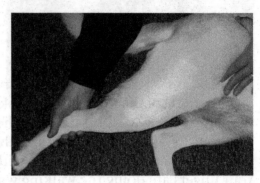

Remember to continue massaging as you ask for the stretch of each hind limb joint. The stretch should be part of the massage continuum rather than a separate component.

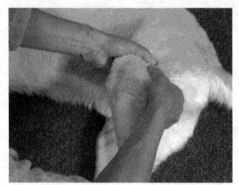

Carefully hold the hind leg at the thigh area **above** the knee (stifle). Be sure to keep the leg **parallel** to the opposite hind leg. While holding the leg, begin to gently move the leg in a small circular pattern. Complete at least five circles in each direction. Return the leg to the normal position.

Begin to use long massage strokes down the front of the thigh. in an attempt to attain a modified "puppy stretch." As the limb relaxes, gently stretch it backward. Stretch only until you feel resistance and STOP. Hold the stretch for 15-20 seconds and gently return the limb to neutral position.

Knee (Stifle) Stretch

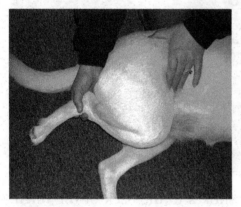

Gently flex the knee and begin moving the ankle bone (hock) toward the pelvic bone beneath the tail. Move the limb slowly while massaging the thigh area. When you feel resistance, STOP. Hold the stretch for 15-20 seconds and gently return the limb 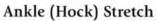 to neutral position.

Ankle (Hock) Stretch

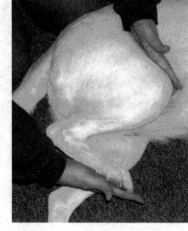

Carefully, hold the bottom of the paw with one hand and the area of the knee (stifle) with the other hand. Slowly, press the paw upward so the top of the paw is moving toward the knee. The hand on the knee stabilizes the limb so the knee and thigh do not move away as you move the paw upward during the stretch. When you feel resistance STOP and hold the stretch for 15-20 seconds. Return the limb to neutral position.

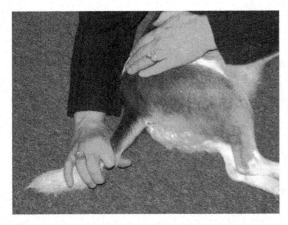

Tail Stretch with Massage

Caution: If your dog does *not* like his tail touched, do not attempt the tail stretches. This will only upset the relaxing effect of the massage. Instead, use a laying on of hands at the tail base and sacral areas.

Now, work your way back to the base of the tail. Rest your hands on the lower sacrum and tail base. Then brush your hands down the tail toward the tip. If your dog does not have a tail, spend some extra time at the tail base using circular and rocking strokes.

Carefully work each vertebra of the tail from the tail base to the end of the tail with gentle squeezing. Return to the tail base and begin to explore each vertebra and space between the vertebrae using tiny circles and thumb strokes. Place one hand at the tail base, which serves as a grounding or contact hand. With the other hand hold the tail about two inches from the tail base and begin a slow, firm, steady pull *directly* backward away from the dog's body. Hold this for 15-20 seconds and then slowly release the tail. Repeat the tail stretch 3-5 times. Return the tail to neutral.

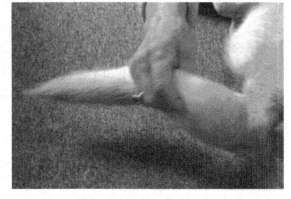

Next, hold the tail approximately 3-4 inches from the tail base and make slow circles with the tail. The movement should originate from the base of the tail. Circle the tail 3-5 times in each direction. After a few sessions, most dogs love the attention given to their tail and greatly enjoy the stretches.

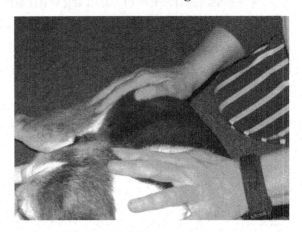

Finishing Touch

Return to light stroking along the back. End the massage by resting one hand at the back of the neck with the other hand rocking the sacrum.

At this point, perhaps a gentle kiss is in order!

The Bullet Version of the Massage Sequence

Happiness is a warm puppy.
— Charles Shultz, *Peanuts*

1. Set the tone.
2. Focus your attention on your dog.
3. Speak softly and think calming thoughts.
4. Place your hands on an area that is most comforting for your dog.
5. Take a few moments to stroke this area.
6. Use long, sweeping strokes from the neck, along the back to the tail base.
7. Massage the face.
8. Massage the base of the ears and along the front edge of the ears.
9. Pull the ear from the base toward the tip, stretching the ear slightly backwards.
10. Massage the top of the neck by squeezing the muscles.
11. Massage with long strokes from the neck to the shoulder.
12. Massage the chest area.
13. Apply slow long strokes from shoulder to the elbow to lower front leg.
14. Combine squeezing, wringing toward the paw.
15. Stretch forelimb forward and backward.
16. Bend the forelimb at the elbow and move the wrist toward the chin.
17. Bend the paw from the wrist toward the underside of the forelimb.
18. Apply long, firm strokes along either side of the back.
19. Roll the skin down entire back.
20. Apply vibration at the sacrum, then use clockwise and counter-clockwise circles.
21. Use circular strokes surrounding the hips.
22. Apply deep circular strokes and compressions on the thigh.
23. Massage the back of the thigh with thumb strokes, with both downward and outward motion.
24. Massage the lower hind leg with squeezing and wringing.
25. Massage the paw and toes. Stretch the toes.
26. Stretch the hind limb, the hip, the knee and the ankle.
27. Use long strokes from the hip to the top of the paw.
28. Massage the tail.
29. Apply tail stretches.
30. Finish with light strokes on the back and gently rock the sacrum.
31. Don't forget the kiss!

CHAPTER SEVEN

FREQUENTLY ASKED QUESTIONS

The best thing about a man is his dog.
— French Proverb

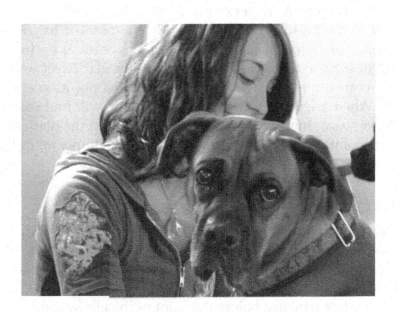

What if your dog moves around during the massage?

Movement is very common when you begin to massage your dog. It is especially common with high energy and smaller dogs.

If your dog moves away and leaves you, it simply means that the massage session is over for him. Begin at his pace with a brief session until he feels more comfortable with the focused touch. If he moves during a session, move with him. You will build more trust by following his lead rather than enforcing how long a session should last. There are other factors to consider.

1. Consider the time of day. For some guardian breeds, such as the Great Pyrenees, dusk is their most active time. This is when the neighborhood may be more active and when predators are in the woods. It is against their nature to settle calmly at dusk. Therefore, this maybe a poor time for massage.

2. Dogs, like people, need your full attention during massage. Disruption and conversation will quickly end a session. Remember to set the tone with as few distractions as possible.

3. Dogs can only tell you they are in pain through their body language and actions. If your dog is in pain from injury or arthritis, massage may cause more discomfort so he will walk away.

4. If your touch is too firm, deep or intense your dog may also walk away. Lighten your touch.

What is a trigger point?

You may have heard this term. A trigger point is a bunching of the muscle tissue, often in the belly or middle of the muscle. Dr. Janet Travell, the pioneer in trigger points, in her book, *Myofascial Pain and Dysfunctions*, defines a trigger point as "a hyper-irritable locus within a taut band of skeletal muscle, located in the muscular tissue and/or its associated fascia." Trigger points are often quite tender. Think of trigger points as energy that becomes congested or stuck. Where trigger points are found, you also will find that the muscle tissue is shortened from overuse or injury. Often a trigger point is not the main area of discomfort. Even though trigger points themselves are tender, they are simply an indication of pain at a nearby location in the area of the trigger point itself.

What does a trigger point feel like?

Trigger points might remind you of the feel of a gummy bear or a jujube just under the skin. Trigger points also can feel like tight strings and tight bands or ropes. They can be quite small or quite large. Many of us have experienced our own trigger points when we feel a knot in our neck or on the top of our shoulders after a stress-filled week. You can easily find a trigger point on your forearm, just below the front of the elbow joint. Using your thumb, press in along the elbow and follow the muscle toward the wrist. In the large part of the muscle, you will likely feel "ropiness" or thickened areas that are tender to the touch. These are trigger points.

How do you find a trigger point on your dog?

Common areas for trigger points are the neck, lower back, behind the shoulder blades and in the middle of large tight muscle areas such as the shoulders and hips. Initially, finding trigger points can be challenging while learning massage. When you regularly massage your dog, you will notice over time when there is a change in the muscle tissue or increased muscle tension. Quite often, those noticeable changes are trigger points. When massaging him, begin with gentle, broad friction strokes to thoroughly warm the area. Once the area is warm, focus on the trigger point itself with compression strokes using the thumb or the palm of your hand, especially in the hip area. Sometimes, trigger points are released in one session. More often, trigger points take time to develop and it takes patience to release them.

How do you distinguish between a trigger point and a tumor?

Sometimes fatty tissue can occur anywhere on a dog's body, and it can feel like a trigger point. Dogs can have a variety of skin tumors both benign and malignant (cancerous). If you think there might be a tumor or questionable growth, consult your veterinarian immediately.

How do you know if you are using the right stroke?

There is no right or wrong stroke. The most important element of any massage is the intention of each stroke and the bonding that is happening during the massage. In general, using any stroke going in the direction of the hair is relaxing for your dog. Look for your dog's signals. Your companion will generally let you know when the stroke does not feel good. Most importantly, he will let you know that you are doing it right by the way he relaxes and sighs.

Practice breathing and relaxing yourself as you do massage and focus on your dog and the signals received during the massage. The problems are generally not about the right stroke but the pressure of the strokes or the rhythm of the massage. Initially, always start with light strokes and later add pressure. Keep your strokes slow, steady and rhythmic. Remember to keep a grounding hand on your dog as you massage. It provides a calming influence.

Can you hurt your dog with any of the described strokes?

No. However, too much pressure can cause soreness and discomfort so remember to use light strokes progressing gradually to deeper or firmer strokes. The wrong rhythm will simply end with your dog moving away.

Can you hurt your dog when doing the stretches?

Yes. When doing stretches take the limb only to the point of early resistance then STOP the stretch. Stretching beyond the point of resistance can result in joint injury. It is also important that you hold the stretch steady without bouncing, pulsing or forcing the limb. Slow, easy and steady movement of a dog's limb, to its early point of resistance, causes no harm.

If you are not a massage therapist, how can you learn this?

No one knows your dog as you do on a day-to-day basis. This makes you the best person to offer massage to your dog. Anyone can learn basic massage techniques.

How is massage different from petting?

The primary difference between massage and petting is intention and focus. Petting is often superficial and mindless and done while watching TV or talking with friends. Massage has the specific intention of relaxation. The muscles, relaxation and what you are feeling beneath your fingers, without outside distraction, are the focus.

Can you do a good massage if you can't remember the muscle names?

Yes, of course. Massage isn't about muscle names; it's about intent, focus and strokes. Knowing the muscle names is useful in understanding areas of stress and when talking to your veterinarian or other health professionals.

How long should a massage last?

The length of massage is totally individual. Factors that govern how much time you spend doing massage are the time available, the size of your dog, your dog's relaxation span and your personal comfort while doing massage. On average, a massage lasts between 10 and 30 minutes. Since you live with your dog, you might focus on one area for just a few minutes or at your leisure take the time to massage the whole body.

If your dog doesn't like a lot of touching, what should you do?

All dogs, like people, need to learn to be touched. First, be sure to set the environment as previously mentioned. While your dog is learning about the touch of massage, begin with short sessions of only a few minutes. There are those areas where your dog likes to be touched such as the ears and under the chin. That is a good place to begin. Leave the tender or uncomfortable areas for another time. Slowly work toward those areas over several days or even weeks. For example, many dogs don't like their paws touched. Don't be discouraged. Be patient, it does take time.

Do you turn your dog over once you complete one side of the dog?

Generally speaking, large dogs are not turned over as it ruins the ambiance of the massage. It can be quite successful to alternate sides from one massage session to another. Some authorities believe that by massaging only one side, the other side of the body is able to learn from this and the whole body then integrates a balance. The benefit of massaging your dog is that you can massage one side one day, another side the next time. A small dog can receive a full-body massage in one session.

If your dog mouths or growls when you give him a massage, what should you do?

Stop the massage at that point. Never put yourself in danger. Usually this is an indication of pain or discomfort. Always listen and be respectful of what your dog is telling you.

Generally, muzzles or other restraints are not recommended as it goes against the intention of relaxation and massage. If you start again, begin with the area where you know your dog likes to be touched.

Is remembering the sequence important?

Yes and no. Dogs prefer little deviation to their routine. The same applies to their massage routine. Begin at the head and cover the entire body first with general strokes, then with deeper more focused strokes. You might want to read the sequence into a recorder so you can listen to it when you are first learning. At some point, you will know the routine and either continue to follow it or improvise, making up your own routine based on your dog's temperament as well as the principles in the book. The sequence you and your dog become comfortable with is the one you should use each time. This allows your dog a comfort zone in anticipating strokes and bodywork. Also, this assures that all areas of the body are routinely covered and you can relax in the process of offering massage.

How do you know if your dog is feeling pain during the massage?

Unlike people who will tell you they feel pain, most dogs because of primal survival instincts don't openly express pain. Signs of pain in dogs are often more subtle. A dog might indicate pain by getting up and moving away, acting extremely playful, twitching his skin, panting, or staring at you. If you have missed any or all of these signals, your dog may mouth your arm or even bite. When you see any of these signs, slow down. Massage the most painful area last using a light touch or laying on of hands.

How do you know how much pressure to use?

Pressure is an individual experience. However, your dog can't "tell" you how much pressure is too much or too little. Practice the massage strokes on your own arm and you will feel the difference between light and heavy pressure.

If your pressure is too much when massaging your dog, he will likely try to get away as the experience won't be pleasant. In general, small dogs tolerate less pressure than large dogs. Finding the right pressure for your dog will take practice. Begin with less pressure and deepen the pressure when you feel both you and your dog are comfortable with the increase. Remember, the primary intention with massage is to relax and enjoy the experience.

Chapter Eight

Common Dog Groups: Their History, Stress Areas and Massage Emphasis

He is loyalty itself. He has taught me the meaning of devotion.
His head on my knee can heal human hurts.

— Gene Hill, "Tears and Laughter"

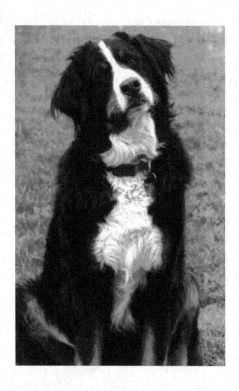

When troubleshooting for trigger points or areas of congested energy, think about your dog's natural tendencies, conformation, habits, activities and anxieties. For example, dogs with short front and hind legs (called achondroplasia) were selectively bred to be dwarfs. These breeds have long backs that cause significant back stress, especially at the lower back area. Also, the forelimbs in these breeds carry eighty percent of the total weight rather than the sixty percent of a normally proportioned dog. This increases the risk of stressors such as arthritis and disc herniations to the back as well as stress to the forelimb joints and muscles.

It is important to consider the purpose for which your dog was bred. This purpose will determine conformation and natural habits. If your dog does not have good conformation for the breed, he is prone to injury. If you have a mixed breed dog, consider your dog's body type and origin.

Dog Group Classifications

Dogs are classified by the American Kennel Club (AKC) into a variety of categories called Groups. Yet, within these categories the breed purpose varies. For example, in the Working Group, the Alaskan Malamute is used to pull heavy sleds and therefore needs muscular hind legs, strong hips and large shoulders. Conversely, the Akita, also part of the Working Group serves to guard. Hence, the Akita's posture is a very upright and sentinel stance. This sentinel stance is very imposing to anyone threatening the domain.

These variations in posture create different stress areas in the body. Due to his structure, the Malamute is more likely to have stress areas and trigger points in the lower back, hips, neck, wrist (carpus), and digits. The Akita, due to the straight hind and forelimbs is prone to knee (stifle) and ankle (hock) problems as well as shoulder injuries. This is because the upright posture allows greater concussive forces throughout the shoulder joints.

By understanding the qualities and conformation strengths of your dog, any weaknesses will become more evident to you. This may help you prevent injuries by not requiring your dog to perform in activities that his conformation is not intended to do or by modifying your expectations. Take extra precautions when performing activities that are not natural for your dog or when he is doing more intense and strenuous activities than his normal routine. Massaging and stretching before and after these activities will decrease chances of injury.

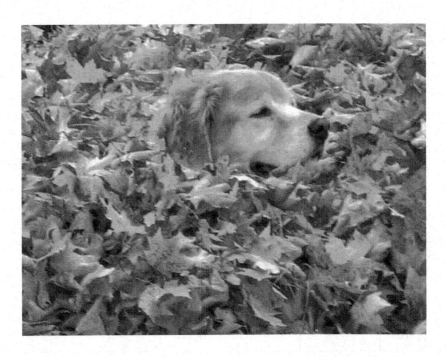

HERDING GROUP

Breed	Heritage/Purpose	Stress Areas	Massage Emphasis
Australian Cattle Dog	Chase & herd cattle	Neck, chest, thighs	Heavy muscled, use deep heavy petrissage, friction, wringing, skin rolling
Bearded Collie	Sheep herding & guarding	Neck, back (slightly long back), tail	Tail pulls, long effleurage to back, skin rolling, neck squeeze
Border Collie	Herding sheep, ducks or geese	Neck, scapula, lower back & ankle (hock)	Massage neck with deep strokes, massage long strokes between scapula & around edges, lower back
Briard	Sheep herding & guardians	Neck, back (slightly long back), tail	Tail pulls, long effleurage to back, skin rolling, neck squeeze
Collie	Sheep herding	Muzzle, face, chest, back, hips	Relax facial muscles with circle strokes around muzzle, deep chest massage, effleurage on the back, petrissage to hips & thighs with gentle stretching
Corgi	Herding sheep & cattle; flushing out ground animals like fox or weasel	Entire forelimbs, shoulder, elbow, wrist (carpus), entire back especially the lower aspect	Massage shoulder muscles with deep strokes, gentle circles along back with special focus on lower back
Old English Sheepdog	Herding sheep & guarding the farm	Chest, lower back, hips/thighs due to its short & compact body, loin area slightly higher than shoulders	Deep chest massage, petrissage thighs, gentle stretching to the hips with small circling strokes, gentle massage to the lower back

HOUND GROUP

Breed	Heritage/Purpose	Stress Areas	Massage Emphasis
Afghan Hound	Sight hunter of large game; some sheep guarding	Neck, face, digits, lower back, tail	Skin rolling to back, relax facial muscles, long strokes to front & back, front paws gently pull toes, tail pull
Basenji	Guide in African forest to warn against danger; hunter of small game	Neck, shoulders, hind limbs (upright posture), tail	Kneading to neck, shoulder & skin roll, tail pull
Basset	Hunting den animals like fox, hare, opossum	Entire back & forelimbs	Skin rolling to back, shoulder kneading, deep forelimbs massage
Beagle	Hunting small game, especially rabbits & quail	Neck, shoulders, entire back & tail	Deep neck massage, skin rolling, tail pull
Blood Hound	Scent hound; rescue work (police/military); unearthing small game	Neck, lower back & tail	Deep neck massage, circles, long strokes, skin roll to back, tail pulls
Borzoi	Hunt rabbits & wolves; Originated in Russia (sight hound)	Narrow deep chest, curved back, increased hind limbs angulation	Deep pectoral/chest massage, long strokes & skin rolling to back, deep massage to thigh & hip area
Scottish Deerhound	Hunt wolves & deer; Originated in Scotland (sight hound)	Smaller button-shaped ear, arched back, tucked tail	Circles to ear base & gentle ear pulls, skin rolling & long strokes to neck/lower back, tail massage, circles & pulls
Foxhound	Hunted foxes along with horses, field hunting (scent hound)	Neck, forelimbs, tail	Deep neck massage, long strokes to forelimbs & shoulder massage, tail pull
Greyhound	Ancient breed used for all types of hunting; fast runner (sight hound)	Arched neck to lower back, tail works as a keel, ears bend toward neck, large hind limbs/thighs, digit injuries from running	Deep neck massage, ear circles at base, ear pulls, deep massage thigh & back, lower limbs, tail massage & gentle tail pull, toe pulls & massage
Otter Hound	Used to hunt otters	Large head, web feet, expressive tail	Head & face massage, paw massage & toe pulls, tail massage & tail pull
Whippet	Hunted rabbits & rats; Great speed, lends toward lure coursing	Deep chest, tucked abdomen & rounded back, tail tucked, digit injuries from running & turning	Deep chest & shoulder massage, long light strokes entire mid & low back, skin rolling, tail massage & pull, paw/toe massage & pull

SPORTING GROUP

Breed	Heritage/Purpose	Stress Areas	Massage Emphasis
Brittany Spaniel	Hunting, pointing & retrieving game	Neck, lower back, tail	Deep neck massage, skin rolling along the back, rocking at the hips, tail pull with circles & squeezes along the tail
Cocker Spaniel	Bird & small game hunter	Neck, low back & hips	Deep neck massage, skin rolling along the back, rocking at the hips
Chesapeake Bay Retriever	Bird hunting; water dog	Neck & shoulders	Deep massage to the neck & shoulders
Clumber Spaniel	Upland hunting	Neck, entire back & forelimbs (slightly long back & heavy body)	Deep neck massage, & skin roll along the back, small circles along either side of the spine, deep massage the shoulders, petrissage & circling around the elbow area, effleurage the forelimbs
Pointers & Setters (English, Irish, Gordon & German)	Hunting birds & game by pointing & marking game	Neck, scapula, muscles of the lower back & tail	Deep massage to neck, circles around scapula, long strokes along back & tail pull
Spaniels – mid-size (Springer, Field, German, Welsh)	Hunting birds & retrieving over difficult terrain	Neck, lower back & hindquarters	Deep massage to neck, long strokes along back, deep massage thighs
Retrievers (Golden, Flat Coat)	Hunting birds both upland & in water	Shoulders, back & hips	Deep massage to shoulders, long strokes & skin roll back, hip stretch
Retrievers (Labrador)	Bird retriever in water & marshes; draw fishing nets, military/police for sniffing purposes; guide dog	Shoulder, back & hips	Deep massage to shoulders, long strokes & skin roll back, hip stretch
Portugese Water Dog	Worked with fishermen pulling nets	Forelimbs, lower back	Long strokes down frontlimbs, skin roll back & tail pull
Weimaraner	Hunting large & small game	Forelimbs, entire back, hips	Long strokes down frontlimbs, skin roll back, circles to hips

WORKING GROUP

Breed	Heritage/Purpose	Stress Areas	Massage Emphasis
Akita	Sentinel; guardian	Shoulder, neck, elbows, knee (stifle), ankle (hock)	Regular gentle range of motion to joints, massage shoulder & elbow areas, neck & hind limbs
Alaskan Malamute	Pull heavy sleds & carts with cargo (mushing)	Hind limbs & lower back (short loin), shoulders, neck, wrist (carpus) & digits if mushing	Hind limbs deep petrissage, lower back, shoulder, neck petrissage if mushing, wrist (carpus) & digit if mushing
Bernese Mountain Dog	Family farm dog; carting; herding/guarding	Back (slightly longer back than tall), Hip/hind limbs (short loin), shoulders & elbows	Circles & effleurage strokes to back, deep petrissage to hind limbs & shoulder, elbow & skin roll to back
Boxer	Hunting, fishing; active in police/military	Chest, neck & hind limbs	Deep petrissage strokes, heavy muscled
Doberman	Active guardian; military/police	Neck, back, hind limbs	Deep petrissage
German Shepard	Active military/police; herding/patrolling sheep; guardian	Low back, hips, hind limbs	Skin rolling & circling along the back, deep petrissage to hind limbs
Great Dane	Boar hunting; guardian	Hind limbs, hips, lower back	Deep petrissage to hind limbs, skin rolling along back
Great Pyrenees	Guarding sheep & goats	Hind limbs, hips, knees (stifle) & ankle (hock), double dew claws, lower back	Deep petrissage to thighs & gentle massage & skin rolling on lower back
Mastiff & Mastiff types	Estate guardians & sentinels	Forelimbs (slightly straight), chest, neck & hindquarters	Deep petrissage (heavy muscled) neck, chest shoulders & hind limbs
Newfoundland	Carting fish to market; lifesaving/ swimming; boating; companion	Hind lilmbs, hips, lower back, shoulders, elbows	Deep petrissage to thighs, massage with circles & skin rolling on back & elbows
Rottweiler	Guard dog for butchers' cattle; military/ police; herding cattle; cart pulling	Neck, hips, hind limbs, shoulders if carting	Deep petrissage to neck, hind limbs & shoulders
St. Bernard	Human rescue	Neck, shoulders, hips & lower back	Deep petrissage to thighs, massage with circles & skin rolling on back
Samoyed	Herding reindeer; pulling light sleds	Back & hind limbs	Skin rolling & long strokes to back, deep massage to thighs & long strokes down hind limbs
Shiba Inu	Flushing/hunting small game	Shoulders, neck, knee (stifle), ankle (hock) (upright posture)	Deep shoulder & neck massage

TOY GROUP

Breed	Heritage/Purpose	Stress Areas	Massage Emphasis
Bichon Frise	Sweet, fun, happy; used in circus & performances	May have hip or knee (stifle) issues, lower back	Skin roll back, deep massage thigh
Brussels Griffon	Ratter in barns	Large chest, straight front, wide muzzle/jaw	Chest, elbow/shoulders, face, jaw
Cavalier King Charles Spaniel	Bird and Small game hunters; kept by English Kings indoors for enjoyment	Straight back	Mid & lower back
Chihuahua	Smallest breed; Religious object of Mexican Indians	Short muzzle & face, straight back, flaring ears	Keep warm during massage, Light strokes to face & muzzle, skin roll back, ear pulls
Italian Greyhound	Owned by European royalty, especially in Italy	Slender, back curves under with tail tuck, narrow chest, straight limbs, chills easily	Skin roll to back, gentle tail pulls, deeper massage to hip areas, keep warm during massage
Lhasa Apso	Guardian with early warning bark at Tibetan monasteries	Slightly long back	Skin rolling & long strokes to back
Maltese	Owned as pets/companions by Royal Court members	Level back & short body	Skin rolling & long strokes to back
Papillon	Owned by Royal Court within the French Court	Body length slightly exceeds height, excellent height/weight ratio, slender legs, high tail carriage	Long strokes forelimbs & hind limbs, Skin roll & long strokes to back
Pekingese	Sacred dog of Tang Dynasty	Slightly bowed forelimbs, high set tail, short muzzle	Face work especially around muzzle, deeper massage to shoulder & forelimbs, skin roll low back
Pomeranian	Companion	Short body, high tail carriage	Skin roll & long strokes to back
Pug	Pet of Tibetan Monks then popularized in Holland & USA as companion dogs	Short muzzle, muscular hind, tight tail	Face work especially muzzle, deep massage to thigh, circles at tailbase
Shih Tzu	Companions to Chinese Court & Tibet	Body length is greater than height, deep chest	Skin roll back, deeper work to chest, gentle pull of digits, massage paws
Yorkshire Terrier	Victorian England; possibly ratter history but mostly companion dogs	Low back	Long strokes from neck to low back

NON-SPORTING GROUP

Breed	Heritage/Purpose	Stress Areas	Massage Emphasis
Bulldog	National symbol of Great Britain; bull fighting/baiting dog through selective breeding; loving companion dogs	Stout, short & bowed limbs, short muzzle	Deep massage neck, shoulders, thighs, forelimbs stretch, gentle circles to face & elbows
Chow Chow	Guard dog; sled dog; hunter	Straight in shoulder & hind limbs with upright posturing, purple tongue	Forelimbs & hind limbs stretches, deep shoulder massage
Dalmation	Coach guardians & carriage dogs; military sentinnel; shepherds; bird dogs & ratters	Fast & strong dog with powerful & slightly arched back, muscular shoulders, long neck	Deep massage neck & back, stretch forelimbs & hind limbs
French Bulldog	Bred initially for fighting; now companion dogs	Short body with slightly rounded back, deep chest, large bat-type ears	Circles to ear base, skin roll & long strokes to lower back, deep chest massage
Finnish Spitz	Hunter of bear, elk & birds; possibly sled pulling	Deep chest, tucked up abdomen, curled tail	Deep chest massage, skin roll & circles tail base
Keeshond	Possibly sled pulling; companions on Dutch Barges; primarily companion dogs	Short compact body, tight tail	Circles & skin roll low back, deep thigh massages, circles at tail base
Poodle 3 sizes Standard, Miniature, Toy	Hunting (water retriever); originated in Germany; popular with European Aristocracy; companion dogs	Square build, short back, deep chest	Standard: deep chest massage & skin roll back Miniature: neck, shoulder, hind lilmbs & lower back, deep massage thigh & shoulder Toy: neck & hind lilmbs, deep massage thigh & shoulder
Schnauzer 3 sizes Giant, Standard, Miniature	Hunter of rats, weasels & water fowl; guard dogs; drover; police dogs; companion dogs	Muscular & squarely built	Giant: deep massage neck, shoulder thigh Standard: skin roll back & deep thigh massage Miniature: deep thigh massage
Shar Pei	Originated in China; guardian of livestock; hunter; companion dogs	Short back slightly concave, many wrinkles, straight shoulder & hind limbs	Deep massage neck skin roll, mid & lower back, stroke face & muzzle, deep massage shoulder & thigh

TERRIER GROUP

Breed	Heritage/Purpose	Stress Areas	Massage Emphasis
Airedale (largest terrier)	Hunted birds & otters	Neck & low back tail base	Deep neck massage, skin rolling to lower back, gentle circles tail base & tail pulls
American Staffordshire Terrier (Pitbull types)	Guard dog, fighting dog in 1800's & now family dog	Very muscular & large muscle groups can become very tight	Very deep massage, kneading, compression, percussion to neck, shoulders & thighs, skin roll entire back
Boston Terrier	Hunted vermin in tunnels of Boston; now family companion dogs	Neck, shoulders, low back	Deep neck & shoulder massage, skin roll back, long effleurage strokes to back
Bull Terrier	Fighting dog in Victorian times, now family dog	Very muscular & large muscle groups can become very tight, knees & hips, expressive upright ears	Very deep massage to neck, shoulders, thighs & hips, gentle circles to ear base
Cairn Terrier	Known from Wizard of Oz (Toto), hunted vermin in stone heaps (Cairn) of Scotland	Upright tail, expressive face & ears	Tail base & low back gentle circles & skin roll, tail pulls, gentle circles to face/muzzle & ear base
Fox Terrier (smooth coat or wire coat)	Hunted foxes	Compact muscular body, shoulders, neck, tail base	Deep massage, neck & shoulders, tail pull & tail circles
Irish Terrier	Working farm dog & guard dog; Originated in Ireland; hunted water fowl & rats; companion	Straight front legs, muscular shoulders	Deep massage neck & shoulders
Kerry Blue Terrier	Working farm dog; guardian of flocks & herds; aid to police; national dog of Ireland	Long neck & head, muscular shoulders, erect tail	Face massage, deep neck & shoulder massage, tail circles
Norfolk and Norwich Terrier	Hunted foxes & rabbits; feisty; companion dogs	Compact, muscular & low built, low back, thighs, shoulder, tail	Deep massage thighs & shoulders, skin roll back, tail circles at base, tail pulls
Scottish Terrier	Hunting den animals (fox, badger & rabbits) Originated in Scotland; companion dogs	Long back, thick tail, short legs	Entire back with skin rolling & effleurage strokes, small circles at tail base & gentle tail pulls
Sealyhaum Terrier	Hunting den animals; originated in England; companion dogs	Similar to Scottish Terrier; long back, thick tail, short legs	Entire back with skin rolling & effleurage strokes, small circles at tail base & gentle tail pulls
Welsh Terrier	Hunter of den animals; worked as hunting hounds in packs; companion dogs	Similar to Airedale Terrier; neck & low back tail base	Deep neck message, skin rolling to lower back, gentle circles tail base & tail pulls
West Highland Terrier	Hunting small game in the lair; now companion dogs	Long back, upright tail, short legs	Entire back skin rolling, tail pulls & tail circles

Workbook Section

1. What was your dog bred to do? (hunt, herd, guard, etc.) If he is a mixed breed, can you isolate one or two breeds your dog most looks like? If you are not certain, obtain a dog book or go online about your dogs breed to learn more about his history.

2. What fun things does your dog like to do (chase balls, bark, run, herd) that mimic his breed?

3. Note the general personality of your dog (i.e. anxious, high energy, mellow) and would this have helped or hindered his original job purpose?

Notes

Glossary of Terms

We give dogs time we can spare, space we can spare and love we can spare.
In return, dogs give us their all. It's the best deal man ever made.

— M. Acklam

Achondroplasia: Short limbed (dwarf)

Adhesions: Bands of fibrous tissue abnormally joined together that often result from inflammation

Agility: A performance sport whereby dogs interact at high speed and encounter obstacles

Anatomy: The structure of an organism or body that includes muscles, bones, organs and blood vessels

Antebrachium: Lower forelimb

Atrophy: Wasting away of muscle tissue

Autonomic Nervous System: The sympathetic and parasympathetic divisions of the nervous system that control functions of the heart, lungs, intestines, glands, the smooth muscles, blood vessels and lymph flow of the body

Body Language: Bodily movements, gestures, facial expressions that express non-verbal communication

Canine Hip Dysplasia (CHD): Malformation of the hip joint common in larger, fast-growing dogs

Carpus: The wrist bones

Cartilage: A tough, elastic tissue

Cervical Vertebrae: The spinal bones of the neck

Compression: In massage, the use of your hand, thumb or elbow to press into muscle tissue to release tightness or spasms

Conformation: Similarities and arrangement of body parts according to a standard

Cruciate Ligament: A cross-shaped band of tough tissue connecting bones in the knee (stifle). In dogs, there is the caudal cruciate ligament and the cranial cruciate ligament that connect the femur (thigh bone) to the tibia (the larger bone of the lower leg). A rupture or tear of the cruciate ligaments is a main cause of hind-limb lameness.

Digitgrade: Walking on toes with the heels not touching the ground as with dogs, cats, horses

Digits: Fingers or toes

Effleurage: Long massage strokes that follow the length of muscle tissue or body part from the neck to the tail. These strokes are relaxing and are also used as transition strokes from one body part to another.

Femur: The long bone from the hip to the knee also known as the thighbone

Forelimb: A front limb such as an arm or foreleg

Friction: A petrissage stroke that involves rubbing or short, quick strokes such as kneading or short alternating thumb strokes either along or across muscle fibers

Geriatric: To grow old

Hamstrings: A group of three muscles in the back of the thighbone from hip to knee that extends the hip joint

Hind limb: A back limb or leg

Hock: The ankle joint in the hind leg

Humerus: The bone of the upper arm or forelimb that extends from the shoulder to the elbow

Kneading: To press, rub or squeeze muscle tissue in massage, a petrissage stroke

Laying on of Hands: Resting hands on a body part for healing or relaxing

Ligaments: A band of tough tissue connecting bone to bone

Massage: To touch by stroking, rubbing and kneading the soft tissue or muscles of the body with the intention to relax, stimulate circulation and/or make the muscles or joints flexible and resilient

Nuchal Ligament: A large ligament over the back or nape of the neck

Oriental Medicine: Healthcare practices of China and the Orient that include acupuncture, herbs and *tui na* massage for prevention and healing of disease

Pastern: The distal part of the foot or paw that includes the metacarpus and metatarsus

Pectoral Muscles: Chest muscles located between the forelimbs and beneath the neck

Percussion: Tapping or striking with hands or fingertips on large muscle areas such as the hips and shoulder muscle groups, best done on larger dogs

Petrissage: Massage strokes that include kneading, compression, squeezing, wringing and skin rolling to improve circulation, eliminate waste and relax

Proprioception: The body's innate ability to perceive itself in space that allows us to jump over objects, walk through doorways or around furniture without hitting objects

Quadriceps: A group of four muscles that form the front of the thigh

Relaxation Response: The ability to learn to relax and respond to relaxing cues such as massage, scents, music

Rocking: A side-to-side rhythmic motion for calming

Sartorius: A narrow muscle of the thigh that helps extend and flex the stifle or knee

Scapula: Triangular bones of the shoulder often called the shoulder blades or wing bones on either side of the upper back

Shaking: A vibration stroke that works with muscle groups instead of one muscle to facilitate relaxation

Skin Rolling: A form of kneading that lifts the skin in order to soften and warm the superficial fascia

Stifle: The knee of a dog

Stress: Mental, physical or emotional tension, pressure, urgency or force

Tapotement: A massage stroke that involves tapping or percussion movements with fingertips or hands

Trapezius: A triangular shaped superficial muscle of the neck and upper back

Trigger Points: A bunching of muscle tissue in response to overuse, repetitive use or injury that often causes pain or discomfort (for example, trigger points found in the trapezius can cause pain in the neck); trigger points feel like a ropiness, tightness, or knot in the muscle tissue

Tui Na: The massage practice in Chinese medicine

Vertebra: Any of the single bones or segments of the spinal column; in dogs, there are 7 cervical (neck) vertebrae; 13 thoracic (mid-back) vertebrae; 7 lumbar (low back); 3 sacral (fused at the top of the hip) vertebrae and 20 (more or less) caudal or coccygeal vertebrae that make up the tail

Wringing: A two-handed stroke done on forelimbs or hind limbs that resembles wringing out a wet towel

Vibration: A back and forth movement such as shaking, trembling or rocking; a stroke used in massage to confuse a muscle into relaxing

About the Authors

Linda Jackson

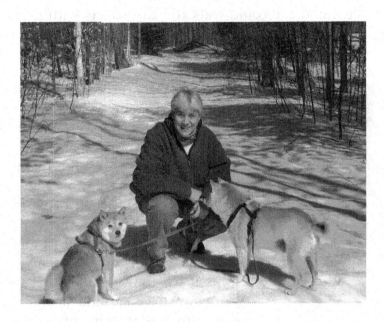

A dog wags its tail with its heart.
— Martin Buxbaum

I began my career as a massage therapist in the 1970s at Kripalu Center in Lenox, Massachusetts. As a founding member of Kripalu Center, I worked with Yogi Amrit Desai in the writing and editing of the original *Kripalu Yoga: Meditation in Motion* book. At Kripalu, I developed programs in massage, meditation, yoga and healthy living. During my fourteen years in residence, I taught weekend programs and month-long trainings to hundreds of people as well as traveled to teach massage and yoga to folks at Kripalu outreach centers around the United States. My private practice began with massage, breath work, yoga and relaxation. In the 1990s I added acupuncture and herbal medicine.

I have Masters Degrees in both Oriental Medicine and in Education. In addition to providing services in my private practice in Great Barrington, Massachusetts, I continue to teach massage and related subjects at Kripalu Center and Berkshire Community College. In 2001, I spent a year at the New England School of Acupuncture to study holistic animal care. Now that I am certified in Holistic Animal Care, I provide services in massage, acupuncture and herbal medicine for both my human and canine clients.

In 1993, I acquired my first dog, a Shiba Inu. Gypsy was the runt of her litter. She was small and very nervous living in the city of Portland, Oregon. My daughter and I worked with her daily to help her adjust to the transition from the country kennel to the bustling city. We tried everything from treats to carrying her to the back yard for exercise and elimination. For weeks, Gypsy would stand and shake. When we took her anywhere in the car, she would immediately urinate on the seat.

At the time, I'd been a massage therapist for over 15 years and knew how massage helps people relax. I decided to try the same strokes and principles with Gypsy. When I massaged her, I focused on my own breathing and relaxing just as I do when massaging clients. I massaged her every chance I could. Gradually, she began to relax. Over several weeks, her shaking diminished and she could walk the city streets with greater ease. Although she never fully adjusted to city life and is now quite happy to be living in the country, she continues to love being massaged.

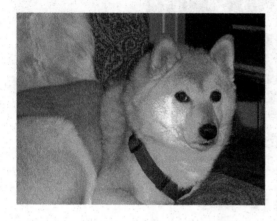

Gypsy, as well as the other two Shiba's in our pack, Romeo and Sachi, continues to receive and benefit from regular massage. The truth is, my dogs don't know the meaning of petting because all touch has become massage. My dogs continue to teach me about temperament, strokes, timing, ambience and scents as well as when or where to stretch them. We enjoy long walks in the woods surrounding our home and in the evenings we curl up with a book or a movie. Having dogs is an integral part of my life, thus it was only natural that they should benefit from my massage and acupuncture training and experience. Now, like me, all of my animals are regular recipients of massage, acupuncture and herbs for health and wellbeing. As a result, we are all healthy and enjoy active lives. Oh, I had also better add, that there is a cat in our household.

I met Jody Chiquoine in early 2000, when she came to me to seek relief from pain that she'd had for years as a result of a serious injury. Soon after her course of treatment, we discovered our mutual love of dogs. Our friendship was forged as we began developing and teaching canine massage to dog owners. Writing this book was a natural outcome of our classes. My hope is that this book will help you discover your love of massaging your dog and deepen the bond you already have with your canine companion!

JODY CHIQUOINE

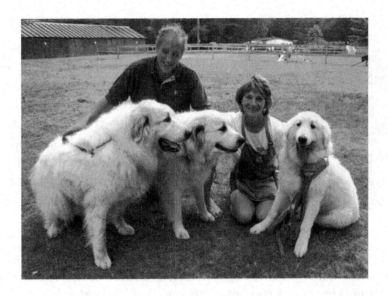

If you don't have a dog, at least one, there is not necessarily anything wrong with you,
but there may be something wrong with your life.

— Roger Caras

In 1999, I started Fitter Critters, a canine rehabilitation and hydrotherapy facility with an indoor swimming pool. I am a Certified Canine Rehabilitation Therapist, and have completed the basic science courses for animal physical therapists sponsored by the American Physical Therapy Associations orthopedic division. In addition, I attend international canine rehabilitation courses and work with canine sports medicine issues including gait analysis. Additionally, I am a member of the American Canine Sports Medicine Association and certified in canine massage.

The myriad of therapy programs in my practice help support the growing needs of both family and performance dogs following illness, injury or surgery. In my work, conditioning, cross-training, fitness and weight loss programs are also individually designed and available. I work closely with all my clients and their veterinarians to provide comprehensive and state of the art canine rehabilitation. For 35 years, I have been a registered nurse and hold a Masters Degree in Nursing as a Family Nurse Practitioner. This profession has provided me with extensive clinical background in rehabilitation, surgery, cancer care and geriatrics.

Also, due to the desire to help owners and dogs, I helped design and introduce the first American Red Cross Pet First Aid course in Berkshire County, Massachusetts and offer instructor courses as well as pet first aid courses to the general public.

I am a founding member of Northeast Pyr Rescue (NEPR), and have served as President to this organization for the past four years. NEPR is a non-profit corporation that serves the needs of lost, abandoned and neglected Great Pyrenees dogs throughout the Northeast.

I live in Lee, Massachusetts with my soulmate and husband, Tim, and three Great Pyrenees, Gaston, Bella and Gentille. We also have our cats, Valentino and Solo, and three pet sheep, Bit-of-Honey, Licorice and Snickers. *All* our family members enjoy massage.

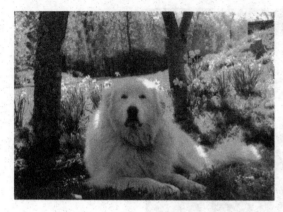

There are deciding moments in our lives. Sometimes those moments are hard to specify and other times the moment is vivid. For me, the day I met Remy was a life-changing moment. He was a one-year-old Great Pyrenees residing on a beat-up sheep farm in Maine. He was born orthopedically crooked—a hind end to make you shudder and he dribbled urine when his bladder was full. When he turned to look at me, I think he actually smiled. I was smitten. Thus we began our lives together.

Remy taught me just about everything I know about canine massage. I massaged his body and stretched his limbs through three reconstructive knee surgeries in 1½ years. Massage wove our life together. He taught me what timing and body rhythm mean, which strokes work best on various muscles, when to do more and when to do less. He learned to both love and demand his daily massage. During these times, I too learned a few things.

Remy taught me that mistakes were OK if the caring intent was right. He taught me to tolerate interruptions because he didn't mind waiting. He taught me that courage is required if one is going to succeed. He taught me to be honest with what I didn't know because then I became more open to greater learning. He taught me to trust my intuition because it often was correct.

I came to the realization that Remy had actually taught me not just about massage but about life itself. Through his eyes, he allowed me to see myself. March 9, 2006, was one of the saddest days of our lives. We had to put our beloved Remy to sleep. He had cancer (lymphoma) but never suffered a single day, which was our gift back to him. Massage was such a part of his life that it seemed natural to be part of his death. When the veterinarian arrived, I began massaging Remy. I stroked and rocked him gently as we talked and he sighed quietly as he settled deeply into the familiar motion. He was given a light sedative and I continued with the touch that was so familiar and calming for him and me. After a while the vet painlessly slipped the needle into his vein. I continued to quietly talk to him as the love in my body, through my hands, rested with him. His slipping away was just a continuum of the life he was used to. Because of what he taught me, I feel that Remy's life continues through my work. What I learned from this incredible dog, I hope to share with you.

Courage does not always roar.
Sometimes courage is the quiet voice at the end of the day saying,
"I will try again tomorrow."

— Edith Wharton

Bibliography

Benson, Herbert. *The Relaxation Response*. Harper Paperbacks, NY, 2000.

Boorer, Wendy and John Holmes. *The Love of Dogs*. Crescent Books, NY, 1974.

Culiffe, Juliette. *The Encyclopedia of Dog Breeds*. Barnes and Noble Publishing, NY, 2005.

Evans, Howard and George Christensen. *Millers Anatomy of The Dog*. Saunders, 2004.

Fisher, Betty and Suzanne Delzio. *So Your Dog's Not Lassie*. Harper Collins, NY, 1998.

Gross, Deborah. *Canine Physical Therapy*. Wizard of Paws, 2002.

Hourdebaigt, Jean-Pierre and Shari Seymour. *Canine Massage*. Howell Books, 1999.

Kainer, Robert and Thomas O'Cracken. *Dog Anatomy: A Coloring Atlas*. Teton New Media, Jackson, Wyoming, 2003.

Marshall Thomas, Elizabeth. *The Social Lives of Dogs*. Simon & Schuster, NY, 2000.

McConnell, Patricia B. *The Other End of the Leash*. Ballantine Books, NY, 2002.

McKay, Pat. *Reigning Cats and Dogs*. 2nd Edition. Oscar Publications, 2004.

Mery, Fernand. *The Life, History & Magic of the Dog*. Madison Square Press, NY, 1968.

Millis, Darryl, David Levine and Robert Taylor. *Canine Rehabilitation & Physical Therapy*. Saunders, 2004

Pugnetti, Gina. *Simon and Schuster's Guide to Dogs*. Simon & Schuster, NY, 1980.

Riegger-Krugh, Cheryl and Darryl Millis. *Basic Science for Animal Physical Therapists*. Printed by the APTA La Crosse, Wisconsin (Orthopedic Section), 2000.

Rugaas, Turid. *On Talking Terms With Dogs: Calming Signals*. Legacy by Mail Inc., 1996.

Yamazaki, Tetsu and Toyoharu Kosima. *Legacy of the Dog*. Yami-Kei Publishers, 1993.

Zink, Christine. *Peak Performance*. Canine Sports Productions, 1997.

Zink, Christine. *Dog Health & Nutrition for Dummies*. Wiley Publishing Inc., NY, 2001

⇥ Notes ⇤

Notes